Teeth questions
What about our teeth?

AF365045

We are learning to take back our own
responsibility for our life, health and actions
and learn to trust the wisdom of the body

2019, Hans Balans

Teeth questions

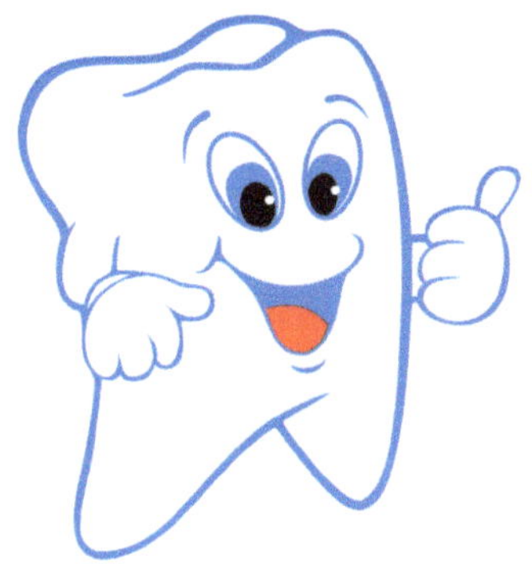

What about our teeth?

Hans Balans

Title: Teeth questions - What about our teeth?
Copyright © Hans Balans 2019
Cover art by Maria Clara Art.Life © 2019
Copyright © Zelfbalans 2019
Published through Ingram Spark
Font: Palatino
ISBN: 978-90-830323-4-4

Genre: Natural healthcare

books@zalfbalans.nl

Index

Introduction

What do we know about our teeth? Are they just a tool for eating and are they made like "rocks"? If so, why do we have 32 of those "rocks" and why is there a system of nerves and blood vessels inside them?

Which visible and invisible systems are connected to our teeth, our jaws, our mouth, our head, etc.?

There are many questions relating to this subject which require a lot of answers.

In this book I try to raise a lot of questions and will answer a few of them using information from different sources. I learned, that when I am able to formulate a question properly, somewhere inside of me I already know the answer. That is the reason why I am able to formulate these questions. When you ask a question thus and trust, the answer will come to you and you might be surprised sometimes which direction the answer comes from.

For me the answers came from scientific papers, dentists, books, channels, internet websites and workshops and sessions with clients.

The insights into the meaning of the teeth in our mouth is mainly of interest to healers, dentists and dentists' organizations.

A lot of new information is coming available nowadays as a result of the investigations of healers, scientists and dentists into the many connections in the body. Most new information comes from people who began to raise questions as well, and began to look outside the existing belief systems for answers, or were able to make new connections using knowledge from other healing modalities.

After a long time of dividing the body in separate parts, each with their own "specialists" attending to these parts; i.e. a cardiologist for you rheart, a pulmonary specialist for you rlungs, ear, nose, and throat specialist, a dentist, etc., many healthcare professionals are now becoming more and more aware of the intricate connections between the different body parts and how they function together as a whole.

It is for example very interesting to look into the dental industry and how it has been completely separated from the healthcare industry and its "specialists", who deal with the rest of the body, in many countries. What are the reasons for this separation, one might ask? The separation is so strong that the teeth are even separated from the jaws in the healthcare industry. They are so closely connected in our body, but treated as completely separate in the healthcare business. I find this very intriguing! It would be similar to looking at flowers separately from the soil in which they grow while gardening. You would need two specialists, one for the soil and one for the flowers! For me this is a good example which confirms how our internal belief systems and programs become manifest in your outside world. Let me explain.

Channeled information about separation

Q: Why do we think that the mouth is separated from the body?

This is a genetic and global issue in the "development" of humans. The mouth is a portal, a connection point with nature. Animals still have this connection, but it is lost in humans. Because we lost

*this connection, we are poisoning ourselves with the stuff we put
in our mouth. Also, the sounds coming from inside aren't divine
frequencies, creating balance with earth and their inhabitants.
The food going into our mouth and the sounds coming out of our
mouth are in disharmony.*

*It already starts with many people right after birth when they
drink artificial milk from other animals or chemically produced
milk instead of breast milk from their own mother, so the
connection with mother (Earth) is degenerated and disconnected.*

My comment:

Maybe there is also a link to babies here. They try to put
everything in their mouth when very young (which is
natural behaviour and something we see in other animals
as well) and make sounds. When they cry it is quite often
because there is a problem in their digestive system. And by
doing so, maybe babies make the exact frequency, necessary
for healing or are telling their mother where the problem is
in their body.

In healthcare the people also think the mouth is separated
from the rest of the body (this is also confirmation for our
beliefs of course).

The same goes for our face and forehead. The boney parts
of our skull have been disconnected and share a connection
with the tectonic plates of mother Earth.

What is so special about the different functions of our mouth?

The dental industry has completely changed over time into an industry of drilling, filling, replacing and invoicing for all kinds of dental problems. It has become mainly mechanical and financial work, which is rather odd when we realize that the parts in our mouth are very sensitive. So, what's going on here?

Our teeth play an important part in our bodily functions as well as our daily life, and have several different functions. You need your teeth in order to be able to eat properly and to make sounds, to talk properly. They can also be seen as part of what makes you beautiful and they give an indication of your health. So, let's treat them as the precious and important things they are with love and care, the way a mother treats her child.

Another issue is the big promotion for "ideal" teeth/smile. According to the industry and healthcare the teeth should be in a specific position in the mouth to "be beautiful". That strong belief from, body shape, clothes, weight, etc. is also influencing the beliefs we have about beautiful teeth.

Is it a good natural feeling when we reconstruct ourselves according outside "rules"?

Are you going to reconstruct your baby child when he/she is imperfect according to those "rules"?

It is a challenge in this society to be the perfect imperfection. That is you! Not the reconstructed version. The unique You is the natural one, with beautiful energy.

Background

Why did I embark upon this project? As an energy healer
I am interested in diseases, dysfunctions on a physical
level, and the connections between the body part which is
identified as the "problem" and the rest of the body.

Before I began to understand energetic healing, I already
had a very keen interest in all the different and intricate
connections in my body and its parts. In fact, I followed
meridian lines and other systems on the body to heal myself
from pains. Since I became aware in 2007 that we are more
than just a physical body, I got even more interested in what
is going on in and around our bodies.

I followed a lot of healing and reading courses, with very
different viewpoints. For me it was important to not just
use one learned technique or modality, but to know what is
behind the technique I learned and why it was working for
many people. What I mean is that each healing "technique"
looks at the body system from a different point of view.
However, the end result is approximately the same for those
different healing techniques. So, I started to "manage" my
body and changed a lot of beliefs and programs in my body
cells and DNA. It has been my experience since that we can
truly heal without pharmaceutical products or surgeries.

Sometime in 2014 I was confronted with a broken tooth and
wanted to repair that in my way. I had read in literature that
it should be possible, because caries can be healed by means
of a change in diet to a more healthy and nutritious diet,
adopting a healthy lifestyle and change our believes. There
was also an article that scientists are experimenting with
laser techniques to activate the healing and (re)growing of
teeth.

So, if that is possible, why is my broken tooth not automatically replaced by a new and healthy one by my body, like my skin, hair and nails are?

In different articles people shared that they grew new teeth, mostly based on a kind of focus or meditation.

I see a lot of people in these changing times and energies who have dental issues, pains or disorders in that area of the mouth.

During my research I already discovered the holistic way of looking at things, i.e. everything is interconnected and working together as a whole. So, the subject is not only the mouth, but the whole body is involved. All the different connections can be confusing when you single out one part of the body to look at. One way of dealing with this amongst scientists is to bring in statistics, simply because they don't understand how it really works. A lot of information is based on statistics and assumptions. However, when a large number of people use these statistical tools and belief the numbers, it becomes a collective belief in our own belief systems.

When I began to dig deeper into this subject, I went from one surprise to the next.

The information in this book is partly based on literature (books, published papers), partly channeled and partly based on my own experience and research. At the back of the book you will find a list of the used literature.

This book is for many people and it is not meant as a story about teeth to read, but to find some information, answers and ideas, which you maybe can use in your life.

Why do we have teeth?

On the internet I found some basic information

Teeth are used for cutting and chewing food. They start the digestive process which gives us the energy we need to live. In the adult human mouth, there are four different types of teeth. They are:

- *Eight chisel shaped incisors used for cutting food*
- *Four pointed canines used for stabbing food*
- *Eight premolars with a bumpy surface, used for chewing food*
- *Twelve molars with a bumpy surface, used for chewing food*

Teeth bite and chew food so that it is small enough to be swallowed. Teeth help you to form words so that you can speak clearly. Have you lost any front teeth yet?

- *Did you find that your words sounded differently for a while?*
- *Maybe you found it hard to say 's'.*
- *Maybe you lisped, eg. "I'd like a thauthage, pleath" instead of "I'd like a sausage please."*

Teeth show when you're happy. People smile when they're happy. If you have nice clean, healthy teeth you have something to be happy about!

Healthy teeth are really important for our overall health. They help us to smile and speak and bite and chew the food we need to sustain ourselves. Milk teeth are the first teeth we get as babies. These teeth start developing before a baby is born and will normally start to come through when an infant is between 6 and 12 months old. When a child reaches the ages of between 5 and 6 their milk teeth should start to gradually fall out with adult teeth growing in shortly after.

People can expect that between the ages of 12 and 14 a child will

have lost all of their baby teeth and these will have now been replaced by a full set of adult teeth.
A full set of adult teeth will amount to 32 teeth in total. This includes the wisdom teeth, which grow in at the back of the mouth. These normally grow in much later and can be expected between the ages of 17 and 21.

So, teeth have more than one function in the mouth. Besides these basic functions I discovered also that teeth provide information, by means of feeling, colour, pain, connection with the jaws, etc. When we learn to feel and watch our teeth, we can learn things about our body and as well as our lives and make changes where necessary. The information from the teeth usually concerns food, health and our interactions with our environment in life. These subjects are all initiated by ourselves, so it is possible to change it.

What is a tooth?

Construction of a tooth

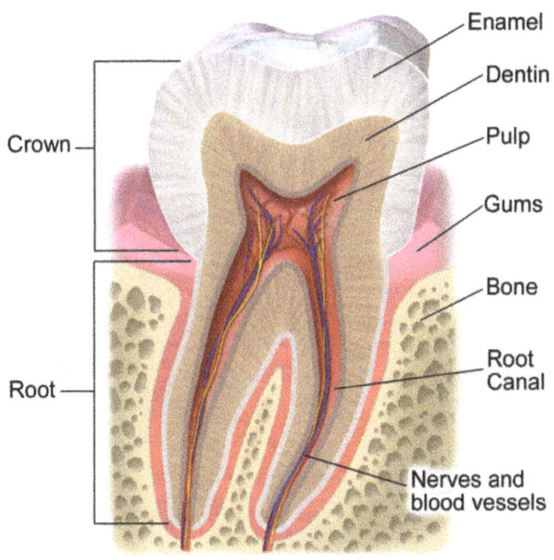

Tooth Anatomy

The tooth has two anatomical parts. The crown of a tooth is that part of the tooth which is covered with enamel and this is the part usually visible in the mouth. The root is the part embedded in the jaw. It anchors the tooth in its bony socket and is normally not visible.

Enamel The hard outer layer of the crown. Enamel is the hardest substance in the body.

Dentine Not as hard as enamel, forms the bulk of the tooth and can be sensitive if the protection of the enamel is lost.

Pulp Soft tissue containing the blood and nerve supply to

the tooth. The pulp extends from the crown to the tip of the root.

Cementum The layer of bone-like tissue covering the root. It is not as hard as enamel.

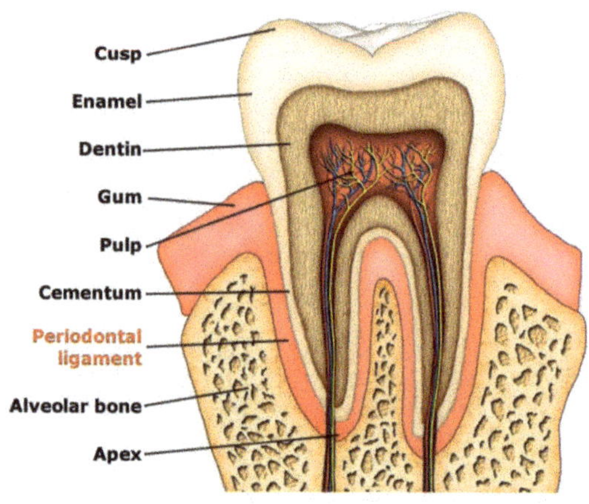

Structures around the tooth

Periodontal ligament: Made up of thousands of fibres which fasten the cementum to the bony socket. These fibres anchor the tooth to the jaw bone and act as shock absorbers for the tooth which is subjected to heavy forces during chewing.

Oral Mucosa: This is the term used to describe the moist tissue that lines the mouth.

Gingivae (gums): Soft tissue that immediately surrounds the teeth and bone. It protects the bone and the roots of the teeth and provides an easily lubricated surface.

Bone: Provides a socket to surround and support the roots of the teeth.

Nerves and blood supply: Each tooth and periodontal ligament has a nerve supply and the teeth are sensitive to a wide variety of stimuli. The blood supply is necessary to maintain the vitality of the tooth.

Creation (or regeneration) of a tooth

During the embryological stage of a child, there are 3 different basic germ layers:

- Ectoderm
- Mesoderm
- Endoderm

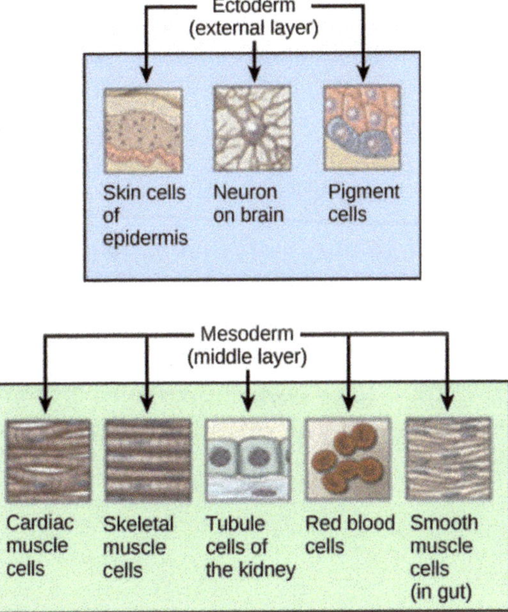

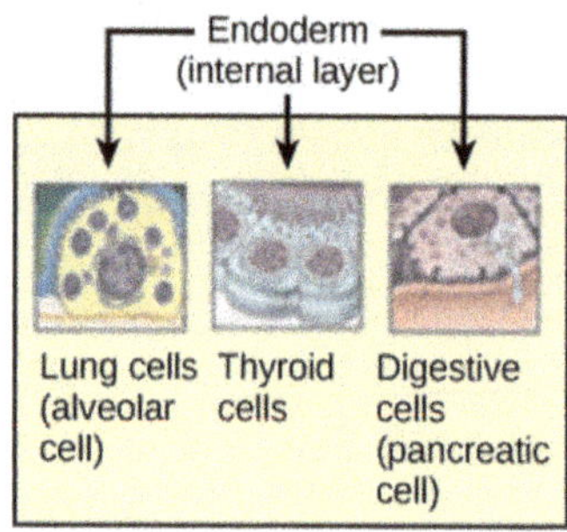

Teeth are built by cells originated from both ectoderm and mesoderm. Enamel is made by ameloblasts from ectoderm and these cells seem not to be present or active after the hard tissue formation is complete. Dentin is produced by odontoblasts derived from ectomesenchyme and these cells continue to exists in the pulp throughout life span.

Important for a healthy tooth is a healthy periodontal ligament. If not, the tooth has a "hard, non flexible" connection with the jaw.

Pulp and Dental regeneration

Regenerative endodontics aims to replace inflamed/necrotic pulp tissues with regenerated pulp-like tissues to revitalize teeth and improve life quality. Stem cells from the apical papilla (SCAP); a unique group of dental stem cells related to developing roots have been shown to be a promising tool for regenerative endodontic procedures and regeneration in general.

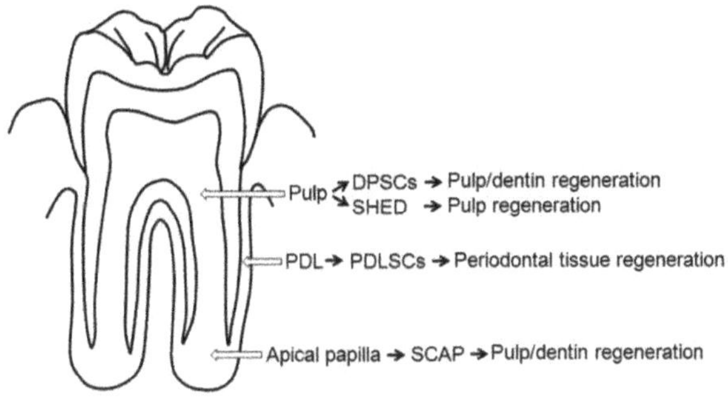

In "Can I get new teeth", later in this book, I will get back to this subject.

Teeth by age

General thoughts about the reasons for humans to have 2 sets of teeth:

Of these 3 tissues (see previous part), the enamel, dentine and cementum are hard tissues, which encase the soft pulp. Note from source on internet: that there are no cells in the enamel and unlike the bone cannot grow or be repaired once damaged.

Therefore, the tooth once formed cannot change in size. But from infancy to adulthood, the body, and with it the structures around the teeth, i.e the maxilla and mandible continue to grow. This leads to increased space in the jaws which cannot be filled by existing teeth.

To make use of the new space formed due to growth of the jaws, the decidious teeth are resorbed, and fall out, and new teeth, bigger in size, which will occupy the increased space erupt. Therefore, we have two sets of teeth- the decidious teeth and succedaneous teeth. Humans have two sets of teeth and are therefore also known as diphyodonts.

Here is the chart of teeth by approximate age of appearance as is usually seen. When we combine the development of chakra's and aura layers in the same first 20 years, you can see interesting combinations. I was informed that these system developments have changed since 2010! I expect more changes in those areas, because children grow up in different ways now.

When we grow up, we pass 3 phases:

- 0 -6 years   milk teeth
- 7 -13 years permanent teeth
- 14-20 years wisdom teeth

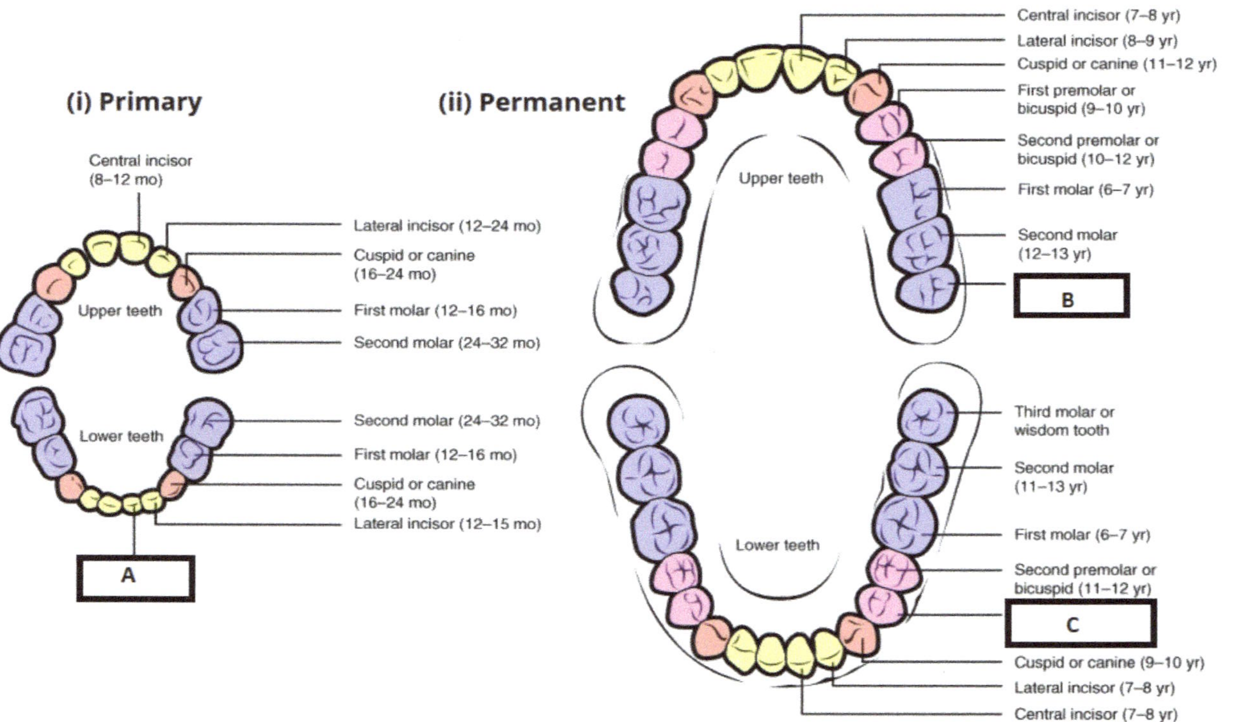

(i) Primary
(ii) Permanent
Central incisor (8–12 mo)
Upper teeth
Lower teeth
Lateral incisor (12–24 mo)
Cuspid or canine (16–24 mo)
First molar (12–16 mo)
Second molar (24–32 mo)
Second molar (24–32 mo)
First molar (12–16 mo)
Cuspid or canine (16–24 mo)
Lateral incisor (12–15 mo)
A
Central incisor (7–8 yr)
Lateral incisor (8–9 yr)
Cuspid or canine (11–12 yr)
First premolar or bicuspid (9–10 yr)
Second premolar or bicuspid (10–12 yr)
First molar (6–7 yr)
Second molar (12–13 yr)
Upper teeth
B
Third molar or wisdom tooth
Second molar (11–13 yr)
First molar (6–7 yr)
Second premolar or bicuspid (11–12 yr)
Lower teeth
C
Cuspid or canine (9–10 yr)
Lateral incisor (7–8 yr)
Central incisor (7–8 yr)

Why do we have so many teeth?

We can ask why we need 32 teeth in our mouth.

Channel on so many teeth

Why do we have 32 separate teeth instead of 2 pieces? Teeth are vital for your systems. You don't know, but there are many interactions between the upper and lower jaw and your teeth. There are vortices between the upper part and the lower part which interact with each other, even when you think! eat or channel. You feel your cheek muscles moving. If it would be one piece in the upper jaw and one piece in the lower jaw, you cannot live so precise and interact with yourself so delicately (sensible? sensitively?). It would be cruder (with only two pieces). Teeth are very strong, but very sensitive in scanning these vortex connections. Yes, if your teeth are not aligned, you won't be aligned, and for example the lower part or upper part will be more dominant, or there will be a mismatch between thinking, intuition and doing. When you develop spiritually you will find a way around the misalignment. With animals it is the same, except the thinking "filter" isn't there or less prominent. They interact naturally based on intuition or reptile brain behaviour. Teeth can be realigned and then processing life and speaking the truth and acting will be realigned. So, you can read jaws better now and solve your own and the issues of others better. Find your way and the meaning of acting in life by reading the aligning of teeth. It will help you in finding your way in life and in knowing how to act.

Artificial teeth are less sensitive, they are more stuck in the jaws. This means the use of jaws will be adapted to a more sensitive movement to adapt in life.

*Aligning teeth will also straightening the teeth to be more
vertically aligned.*

*Dis-alignment is very good for certain experiences of materials,
stars, species (humans). But it can be realigned by recognizing
and solving issues in awareness. These consciousness fields can be
changed by changing believes and by releasing or accepting fears.
But doing/acting is important. Acting is aligning and learning
with source.*

What is the relation between body and teeth?

The body and the mind can not be separated. Neither can all of the many processes that happen in the body each and every second. All of the hormones and neurotransmitters of the body are in constant communication with each other, and the body is constantly adjusting for changes in energy supply and demand, as well as anything it experiences in the environment. Because of this, a holistic approach is the only way to fully deal with any imbalances in the body which lie beneath symptoms and, ultimately, disease.

A holistic approach considers all aspects of a person's health and recognizes how these are all connected. There are many ways that the body can get thrown off balance, and different people are susceptible to developing different kinds of symptoms. The entirety of systems and organs of the body do not operate independently of each other, therefore what happens in your gut affects your cardiovascular system, your adrenal system, your brain, your hormones, your immune system, etc.

We gradually see an increase in a more holistic approach in dentistry develop over the last years, but this approach is quite often based solely on the meridian system. Is that all there is? Let's look at it and see what other connections there are which influence the health of our teeth.

Connections from and to the teeth

1. Physical direct connections

The first connection I looked at, were the direct connections of skeleton and the muscles.

The connections in our body skeleton are very interesting. Everything is connected and when one part moves, other parts move as well because of this initial movement. This is also the case with initial static postures. If a particular body part is held in a certain position, you can sense it in other parts as well. So, if we continue to put a certain body part in a particular static position over and over again, for whatever reason, the complete body takes a certain posture. This is how we observe people, their posture and their energy field, and it will probably not come as a surprise to you to know that those are related. The body reflects (or shows) the energy field. The energy field as mentioned here is the innate field, which you also can observe in many other ways, like for example the aura field.

Even the movement of the skull bones makes a difference in total body posture!

There is an interaction between the area under the lower jaw and the skeleton, guided by the floating throat (Hyoid) bone. See picture.

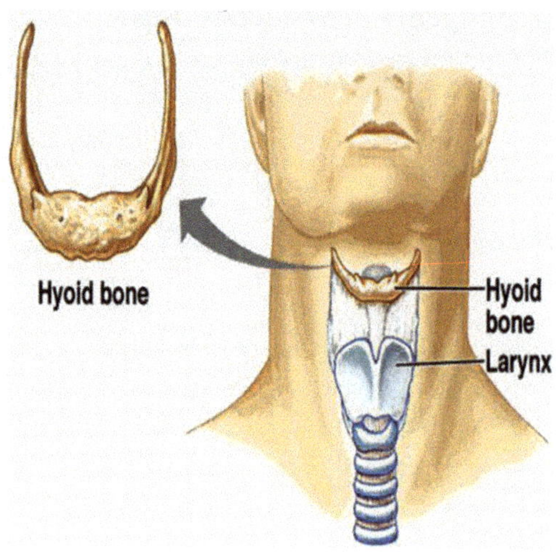

This bone is by muscles connected to the skeleton, shoulders and lower jaw.

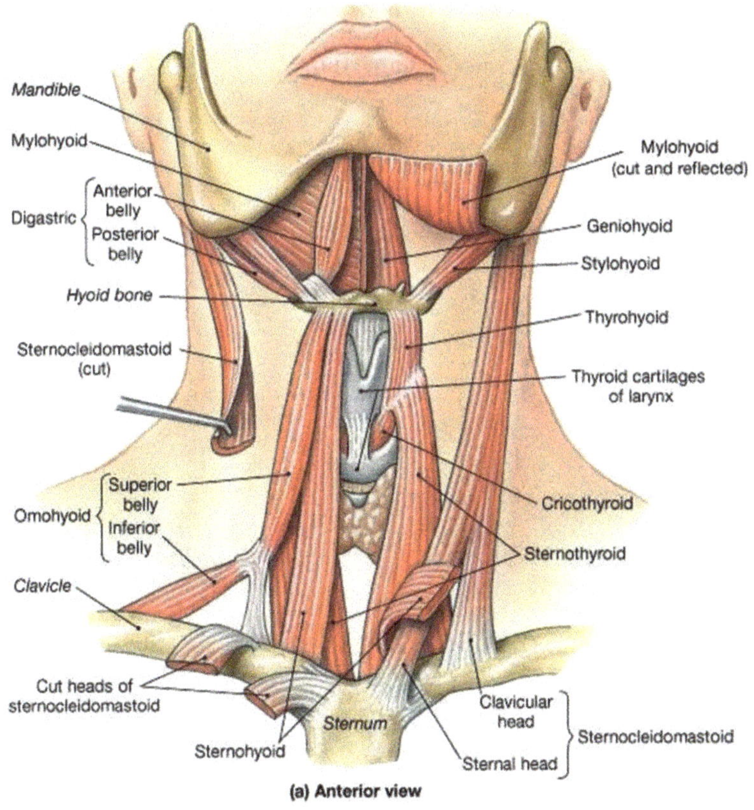

(a) Anterior view

The upper jaw is connected to the skull by boney parts. These boney parts of the skull are also flexible in relation to each other and separated by soft tissue, which contains bloodvessels and nerves, etc.

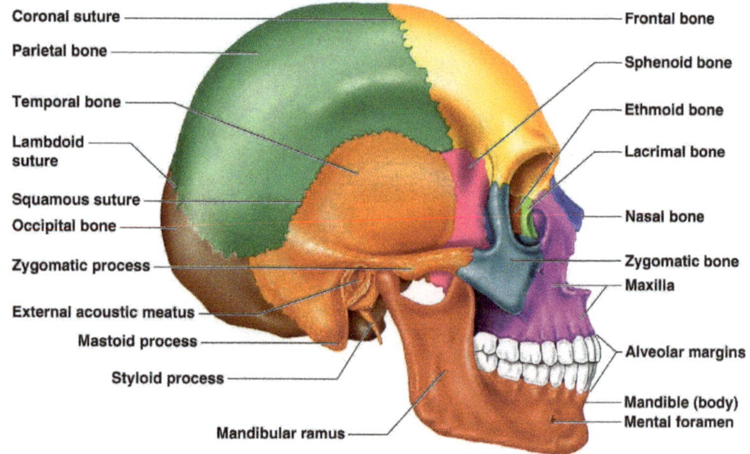

The connection of the lower jaw to the upper jaw is by far the most complex joint in the body, the temporomandibular joint (TMJ).

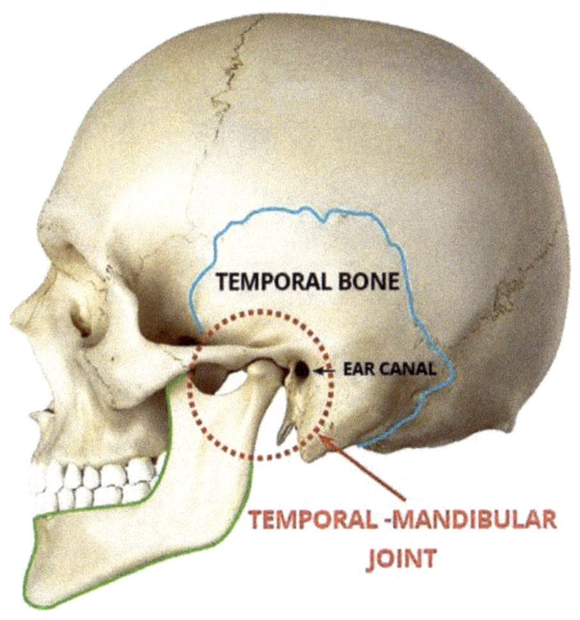

The TMJ can move in many directions. This flexibility also makes it vulnerable. And yes, many people suffer from a disorder affecting the TMJ, called TMJD (Temporomandibular disorder). There is a specific chapter on this subject further along in this book.

2. Nerve system connections

The next interesting part of our face is the trigeminal nerve.

This Nerve is connected to upper and lower jaw, face and the teeth.

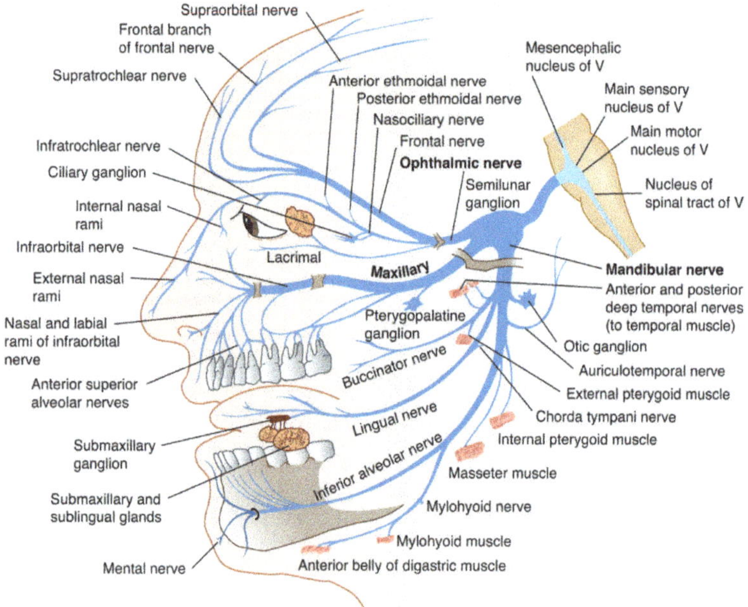

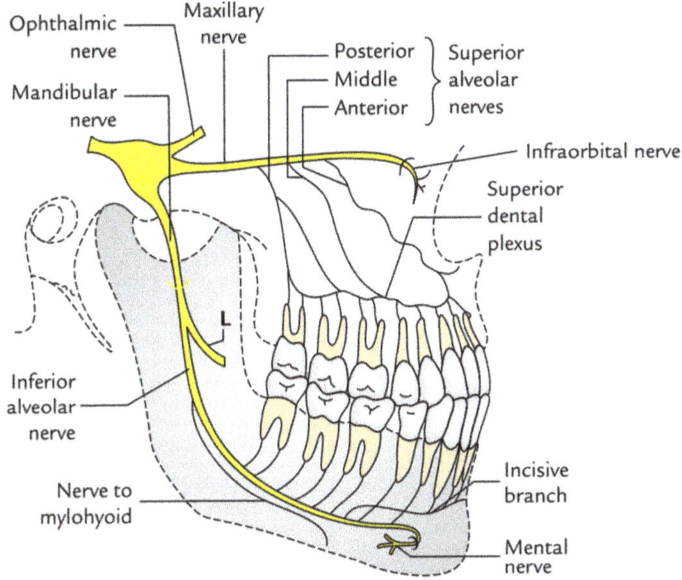

On the other side of the nerve it is closely connected to the parasympathetic and sympathetic nervous system in the neck, where these nervous systems come close together. And it can pick up signals from the spinale nerves in the part where they cross.

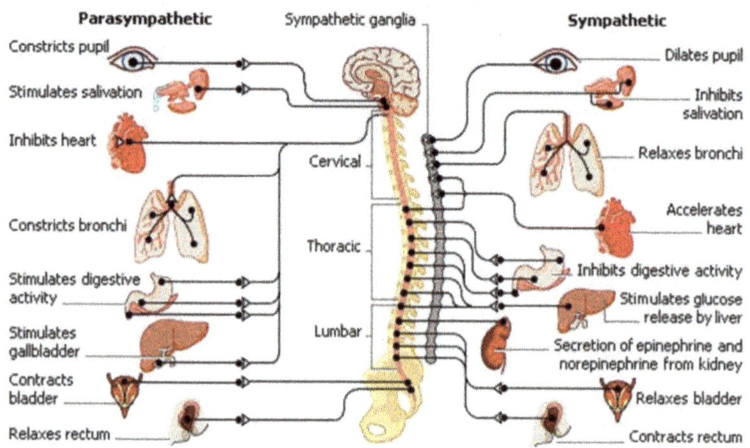

The spinal cord will give off alarms and other signals indicating dysfunctions in its system in relation to many body parts and organs.

So, the trigeminal nerve interacts with all organs and their signals! And it gives signals to the muscles and skin functions of your face as well. This means that the expression of the face is influenced (or controlled) by this nerve too. Everything is connected.

3. Hormones and blood system

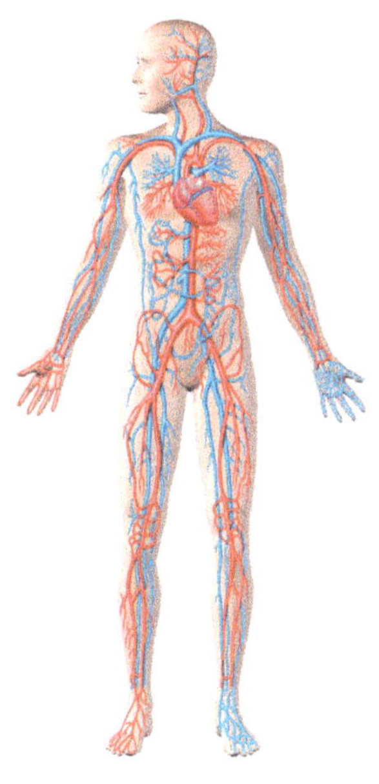

The blood circulatory system has connections inside the teeth and in all other parts of the body too. So, a lot of information is circulating in the blood, like hormones, minerals, vitamins, blood cells, etc.

This includes information from "problems", like disease, disorder, etc. Not only does this information circulate through the body, it can also influence teeth, or the other way around, teeth problems can influence other body parts by means of the blood and hormone system.

The transportation of minerals and vitamins needed to feed the jaws and teeth is also very important in keeping the teeth healthy and strong.

We will talk about these minerals and vitamins later, but I think it is already important to mention here that we need the right minerals and vitamins in circulation, so the food we eat and what we drink is very important for the health of our body and teeth.

4. Meridiane system connections

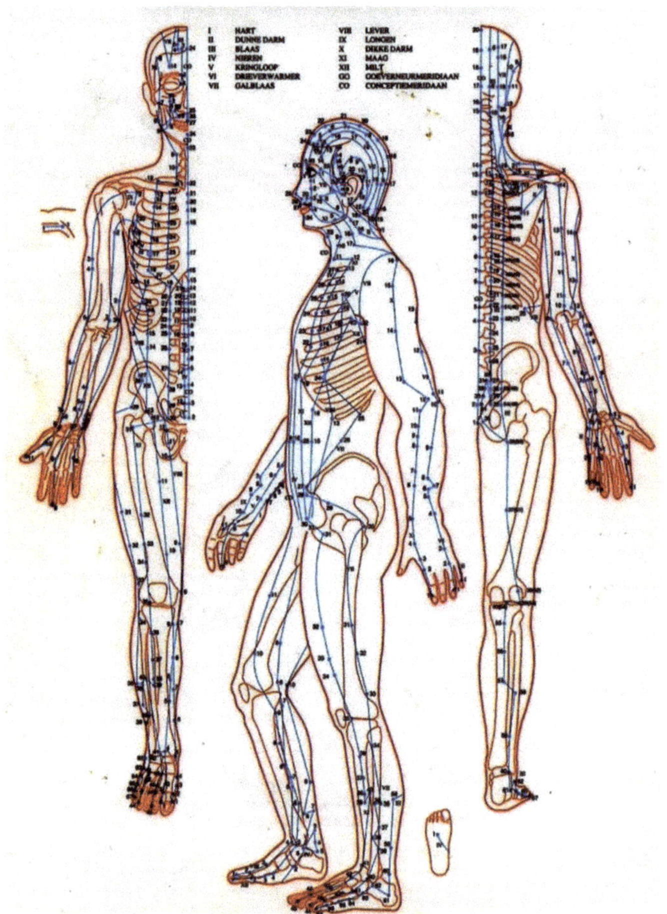

The meridian system is very interesting.

In dentistry there is currently a trend to look at the meridians for healing. It is definitely a good start to look at teeth from a different perspective in a more holistic way.

The basic meridian charts find their origins mainly in eastern countries according to literature.

If you look at the standard charts, which most people use, they do not show very many meridians going directly to the mouth and ear. But if you look at the detailed charts people use in healing, you will see it is much more complex. See the below pictures of the mouth and ear. So, it seems that there are more meridian connections. Maybe the meridian system looks more like the root system of a tree with main roots and many smaller roots spreading in the earth?

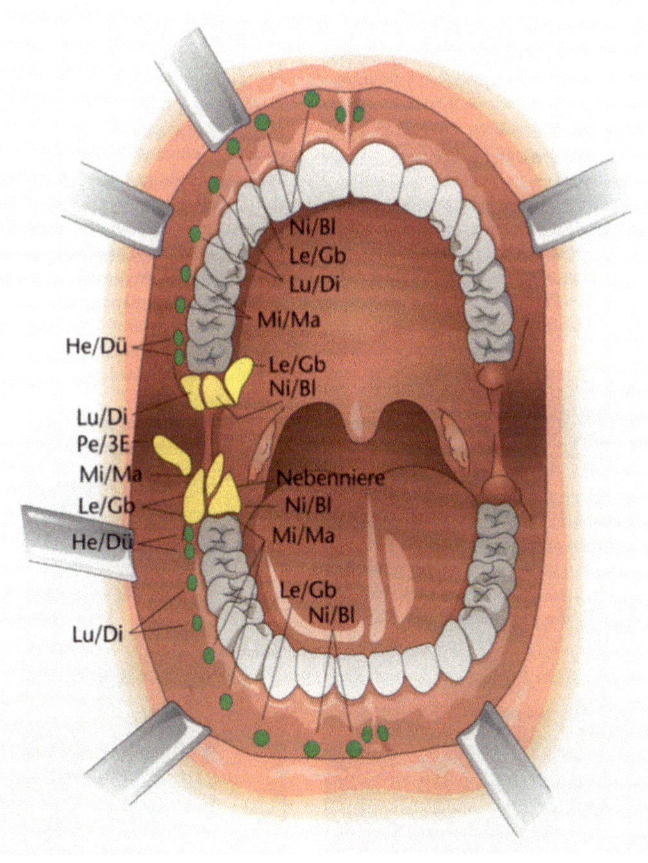

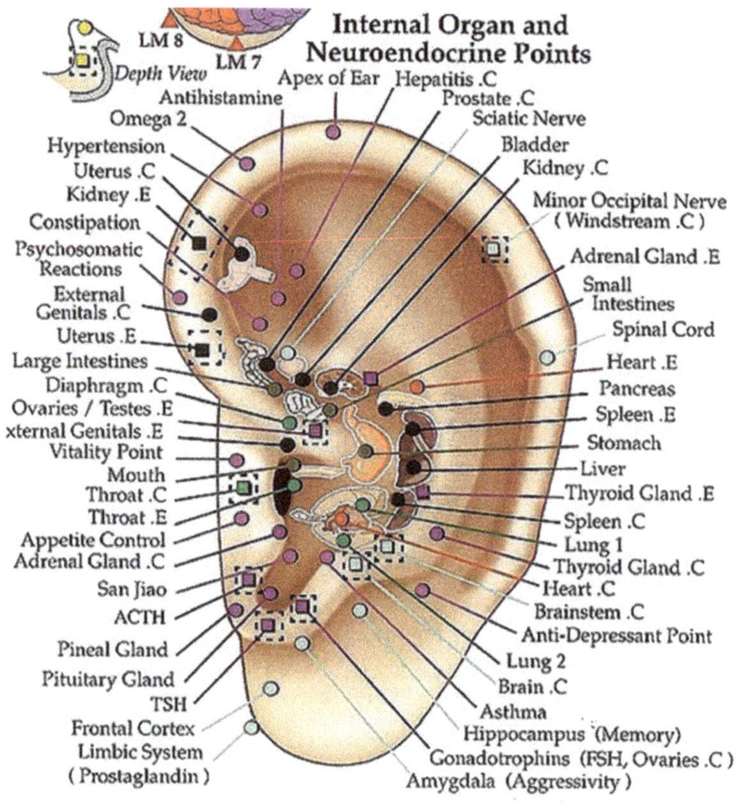

Channel on meridians and body movement

How are meridians connected to body movement?

Meridians are flowing in and out through and out-in the body. They are in contact with the surroundings, like the earth, air, sun, etc. The information gathered from the surroundings is necessary for the entire system of the body. for example, the hand meridians are for info to and from the hand's movement. If natural movement is blocked, the meridian will block too. What are natural movements and what are forced movements? What is holding you

38

back from (natural) movements? What is the information you
are resisting or what is it you naturally do? Yes, the meridians
are linked with movements of organs, hands, feet, legs, etc. In a
healthy system everything is in constant flux. When movement
stops, something in your system blocks too. The information from
meridians is then blocked as well. Blocked energy hurts. Therefore,
you have to find the cause of the blockage of movement. Where
does it hurt and what would that organ or body part really want to
do? Even when sitting or sleeping everything moves. Think about
that.

What is keeping you from a natural posture or movement. Talk
like you talk to me to the body parts or hurt with the same energy.
For healing by movement, you really need to feel/talk with your
body and ask it how it wants to be moved. Yes, Moshe Feldenkrais
understood how to intuitively feel what movements to make, just
like you heal with Transhealing. It's all about trust in what you
do. Do not block your movements. Understand that the body
knows how it is designed to have posture and movement. That
original blueprint of **yourself** is changed by **yourself** to show
yourself how you are doing. Find the natural posture and way to
move based on your blueprint and solve the issues which caused
you to change it and keep practising the MF movements and really
feel it and **remember** that feeling. So, you overwrite it with the
original program/blueprint. No, you cannot remove in one shot by
mental! Movement is feeling, is meridian info flow.

Any questions? Yes, about the function of the meridians in our
arms.

Arms are part of your posture and doing things. But **how** are
you using your arms, when you do things? How does it feel? Be
aware. Posture is confidence, be aware of how you let your arms
"hang" and feel confident. You can either let them "hang" or move
them. You can play in front of a mirror and **remember (= fix)** that
feeling.

So enjoy!

5. Lymphatic system connections

Like the blood circulatory system, the lymphatic system has a wide network reaching all parts of the body. Information from and to the mouth is also moving through this system and to other parts of the body.

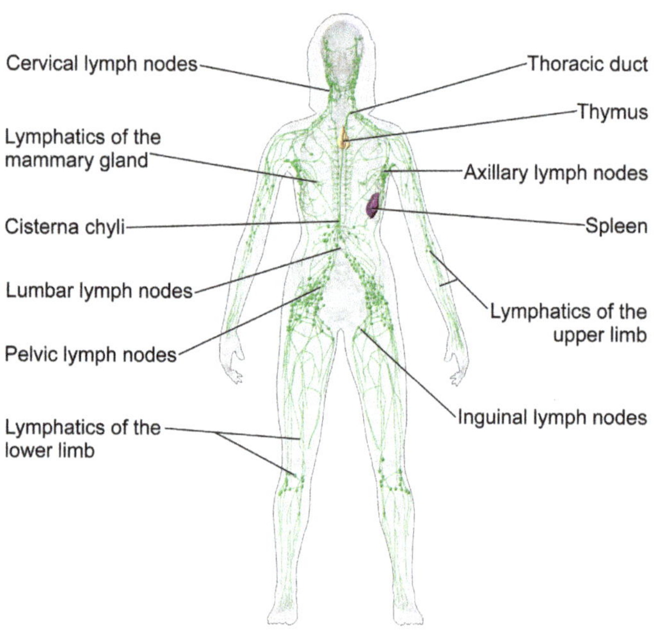

6. Light and Biophotons and water connections

Science is for a long time searching for the meaning of light in and around cells. What is the meaning, function, activity of light? Is it coordinating, communicating between cells, or...

Recent alternative research found similar results in relation to water.

In one of the channels this was confirmed to me. Water and light in the body have sometimes similar functions and interactions.

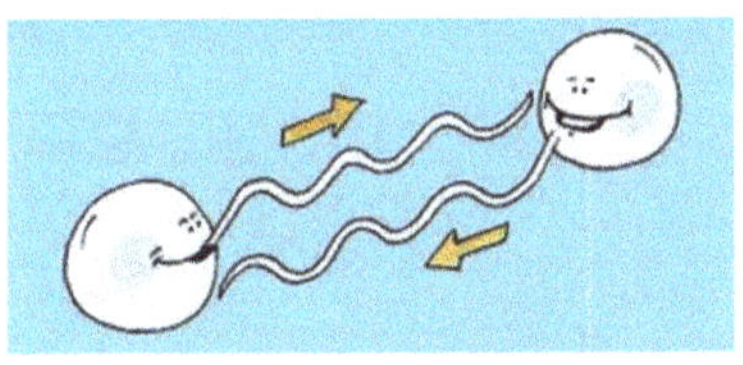

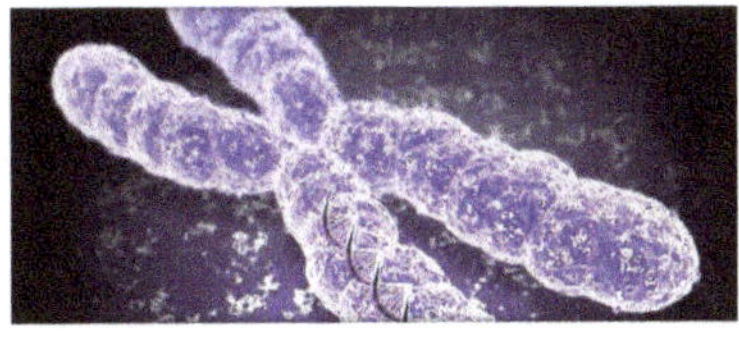

Light and water coordinating and informing so many processes, it is very complex and simple! Sometimes it looks like light = water.... or water is compressed light.

Scientists also found that light is forming structures in cells.

Because all the organs, nerves, muscles, etc. have cells, the light seems to control or at least influence many systems in the body. Also, our circadian clocks (for repeating body systems) are working with light systems.

In this subject we can make the connection with coherent systems and the coherence of light. This coherence system is explained later in this book.

Conclusion of this subject is that communication in the body is also happening by light and water. And light is very fast!

Channel on light and body

What is light power and what is the connection between love and light? I'm talking to you about light, frequencies and crystals. Crystals are light and you are crystals, stars, light. You all radiate frequencies, light "energy" and love. Higher love is a form of light for the higher heart. Not to be confused with human heart "love". Light is always present, but you want to hide it as humans. It is rather funny to see you hide yourself like a kid, but everybody can see you. Why do you hide?

You think that a stronger light does not exist. At least that is your experience. You allow other (higher) frequencies to pass through your light filters. Yes, that's how you create yourself and your view. Seen through these filters, light "looks" different. And light can not always be seen. Do you "see" your light like the light from a lamp? No, because it is energy, a frequency in consciousness fields, so there is your connection to love and light. The frequency ranges of consciousness fields of love are absent, thrown out of balance or seen as duality as a result of your filters. When seen as duality you "see" more frequencies instead of only one at the same time, which creates imbalance. Sometimes it looks balanced, but it is not. Pure "light" is what you would call power, that is pure light from one tone, one source. You know the expression "speaking with a double tongue"? You hear duality! People sense the double flow, the double creation. So, if you allow all frequencies from pure source you will feel "power", power of light. But in fact, it is unfiltered pure light that you feel. Be the source, remove or adjust your filters. Just like clear water. You can see much more in pure source water and you can feel the pure vibration of source water. No filters on troubled views (unclear where to go), you see? The more you allow pure light in, the more clearly you can see and know where to go in your life. Make your light pure, clear. Then you see, know and understand things better. The more unclear the view, the more humans are struggling with questions in relation to where they are and what to do. They don't understand what is going on anymore...

Helping, serving others is opening them up for pure light. You feel lighter. Do you understand?

So that's all, so simple. Questions?

What is the relation of light and health, vitality and beauty?

You know about beautiful crystals, their frequencies and pure light. You are a crystal, a star. So, your cells are also crystals; light in a moving flexible form in your belief. So, the purer light, the "healthier" the cells in your body will be. That is healing. Healing is light, it is removing filters for pure light. You are pure light so you understand now.

What about getting older?

What you call getting older is in fact not so. You get wiser and you may have changed and removed several filters necessary for your purpose and experience. The light reflects back to source(reflection) from your crystalline radiation and the cycles in your experiences. The resonance in the collective cycles and experiences calls you home but now you can stay on the basis of free will and change your contract frequencies with the group consciousness frequencies and in doing so immediately change your light game which gives you the choice to go on or go back. That process of reflecting light to and from source is also part of your experience and you can choose to stop and let your body close down slower, or stop light and shining and return faster. This is a sign of strength with that experience instead of instantly going back. In the past elderly people were honoured for this. Because of their wisdom and knowledge of their experience. You don't understand that anymore. That's why you asked the question. Now a lot of elderly people experience alone time to learn and honour themselves. You see every period has its own challenges.

See you next time in light.

7. Consciousness fields connections

The last layer in and around the body which can influence and interact with teeth is the consciousness field of every cell, organ and body.

Every cell has a consciousness field which interacts without spatial limits with other consciousness fields at a speed which is much faster than light. It looks like consciousness is travelling without time, it is in the present moment.

Although it is confirmed by science, this is a very complex subject to clarify in one chapter of this book. It is my daily work to interact with these fields and I know it is working.

It is for the purpose, namely the connections to and from teeth, not important to know exactly how it works. It suffices to know that it exists and works.

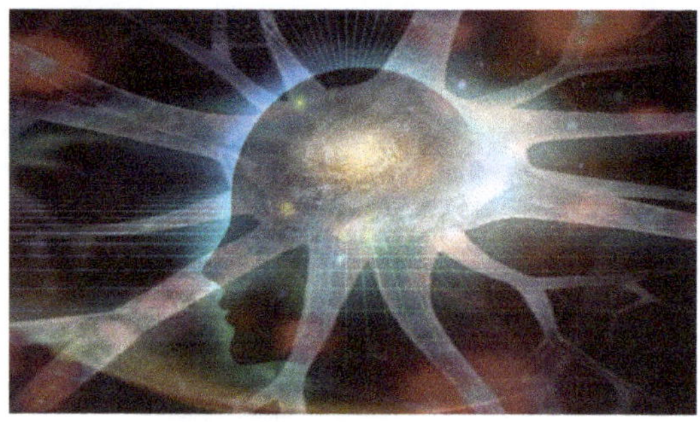

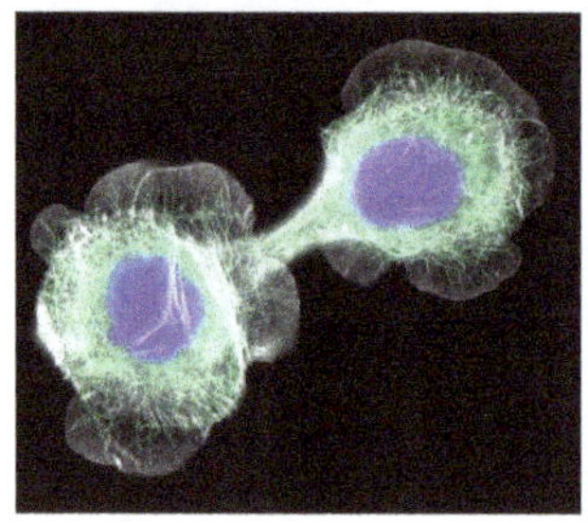

All the 7 layers of connections

there are more than 7 layers of connections in and around the body which influence the teeth and body in both directions. So, are teeth still like small rocks in our mouth?

There is a lot more going on than we can imagine. What is important however is that we realise our body is a complex system. Or… is it perhaps just very simple?

When we use our senses like seeing, hearing, feeling, tasting, smelling, more on a daily basis, we get a lot of information from the body. We can compare our sensations from one day to another and discover little changes. In my opinion this is the most important part of life many of us have forgotten. But it is not too late to change and learn.

On top of these senses mentioned here, there is also an important tool, integrated in our bodies, which we can use to ask the body questions! With kinesiology we can ask the body and its systems questions. This is an amazing built-in tool and everybody can remember or learn how to use that. For example, we can ask the body what it needs in terms of food, vitamins, minerals, etc. We can test whether food products in shops are good or harmful for the body. We can test whether technical equipment such as cell phones, wifi, electronics, motors, and the like are harmful for our systems, or not. So, my advice to you would be to go to the nearest workshops where they can teach you this simple tool to test yourself.

Why are there so many problems?

Human beings have shifted their focus on economy, money and technical objects and have forgotten the part about life, nature, earth and universes. The people we call (ab)originals still remember many things about original life on earth. They have knowledge from the past. I come back to this subject in the paragraph about food.

Just like everybody else, dentists are also focussed on making a living and earning money. I notice a shift in recent years towards being more of service instead of making more money. Some follow that and some refuse. It is our choice which dentist we choose.

The other problem is the separation of everything. We split the body in many small parts to focus on when we have a "problem". In this way we created "specialized" people, earning money by looking at a little part of the body. In the past paragraph we discovered the many connections, so the original holistic view slipped away in this process of separation. But there is good news, we start to remember this way of looking at the whole body and... beyond.

The many teeth "problems" are there, because of our present way of looking at life, the food we eat, the emphasis on making money, our focus on a little part of a "problem" and because we forget when the "problem" started. The cause of the "problem" is more interesting then the analysis of the "problem".

In this book I give some guidelines how to change things in your lives and heal, recover and revitalise your teeth. It can help you in more ways. You have healthy teeth, you feel better and you get information what is going on in your life. So, you can do things differently if you like to change.

What is relation between teeth and food?

Based on published research, the numbers of cavities have increased dramatically over the past years, particularly in children. This is in contradiction with increased dental hygiene.

The increase in bad nutrition is however in line with the dental problems, so there is something to win very easily by just eating good food (when available!).

Another interesting research result shows that older people (>65) have better teeth conditions than younger adult people. The number of lost teeth is much higher in younger adults than older people. So, what is the secret? Health, happiness, less stress, food and so on?

Dr Price already investigated in the 1920 -1930 's the effect of changing diets on teeth. His results were very interesting. And he did research in many countries all over the world. Good nutrition can not heal damaged hard tooth material, but it can prevent and heal cavities. That is a big step in keeping healthy teeth.

You can read more about these investigations and results in his papers and on the website of Dr. Price. Some interesting notes from that public material:

After spending several years approaching this problem by both clinical and laboratory research methods, he interpreted the accumulating evidence as strongly indicating the absence of some essential factors from our modern program, rather than the presence of injurious factors. These investigations have been made among the following primitive racial stocks including both isolated and modernized groups: the Swiss of Switzerland, the Gaelics in the Outer and Inner Hebrides, the Eskimos of Alaska, the Indians in the far North, West and Central Canada, Western United States and Florida, the Melanesians and Polynesians on eight archipelagos of the Southern Pacific, tribes in eastern and central Africa, the Aborigines of Australia, Malay tribes on islands north of Australia, the Maori of New Zealand and the ancient civilizations and their descendants in Peru both along the coast and in the Sierras, also in the Amazon Basin. Where available the modernized whites in these communities also were studied. There have been many important unexpected developments in these investigations. While a primary quest was to find the cause of tooth decay which was established quite readily as being controlled directly by nutrition, it rapidly became apparent that a chain of disturbances developed in these various primitive racial stocks starting even in the first generation after the adoption of the modernized diet and rapidly increased in severity with expressions quite constantly like the characteristic degenerative processes of our modern civilization of America and Europe. While tooth decay has proved to be almost entirely a matter of the nutrition of the individual at the time and prior to the activity of that disease, a group of affections have expressed themselves in physical form.

Dr Price's conclusion was that nutrition and way of living was the main cause of dental problems.

We can discuss many subjects in relation to the nutrition of indigenous and ancient people and modern nutrition, but for me there are a few aspects which are important in the light of nutrition:

- Minerals, fats and vitamins, like Calcium, Phosphor, K2, D (Codfish) fish oil, D3, B1, A, C, B12…

- Taking care in the morning and cleaning in evening.

Based on the investigations of Dr. Price vitamine K2 was
recently discovered by Ken Southward as the "X-factor"
of Dr Price. Vitamine B12 is more related to the gums and
general health.

Food is one of the connections with our environment. *"We
are what we eat"*. The food we eat influences our entire
system, even our cell functions and the health of our cells.
The RNA from our DNA creates enzymes to determine
the function of the cell. Healthy food with all needed
ingredients creates healthy cells and a healthy shining body.
Even the structure is determined by our RNA creation, so
we can influence that with food. Other influences are genetic
influences and our thoughts! It is this combination which
makes you healthy and vital. If your thoughts are focussed
on being happy and eating for a healthy body you recreate
your body in a healthy and vital way.

Also, the understanding that we are part of this planet, this
universe is very important. We are interconnected with
all beings, planet and stars. There is a saying: *"we are made
from the stars"* or *"starseeds"*. In fact, this is true. We are
interconnected with the stars and influenced by the stars in
our daily life. We like to read astrological information about
our lives, our self and our future, not?

When you know where your food is coming from and what
its function is for your body there is a way of "controlling"
or "mastering" your body and body systems. We need
to understandthe system and be grateful that we are part
of it. Healthy food also means avoiding toxins. That is
also a problem these days with all the processed foods.
Gluten for example is not an ingredient we need to replace.
The problem with gluten is that it is just poisoned food.
Pesticides, GMO, etc. are unnatural and only used because

they are believed to enhance production, as a means to control nature, and symptoms of the desire for speed in life and of course the desire for more money.

Every person needs to check what their body needs; food is personal! There are general rules, but for the rest feel what is good and what your body needs. You can talk to your body about this. I discussed this before, learn kinesiology and play with it. When you use it daily your system already informs you, before you ask.

There are several suggestions in literature for healthy nutrition. Some suggestions from the authors:

Change your diet

Diet is very personal, so everybody should test for the right diet and healing.

What is missing in our food program for healthy teeth?

- K2 and D3, Phosphor, Calcium and B1
- Oil for mouth oilpulling in the morning, like Sesame oil, or Aman Prana menta mouth oil or coconut oil.
- Vitamin A and D, the best form from cod liver oil, fermented.
- Vitamin C

What should be avoided or replaced (if you think your body needs it)

- Artificial sugars and sweeteners, ALL of them!
- Cow/animal milk, except some raw milk products.
- Microwave food.
- Whole grains!
- Processed food in general.

Processed milk, like pasteurization, destroys components needed to absorb Calcium, Phosphorus, probiotics and vitamins from the milk. So, it loses its function and the side effects are worse, like for example poisoning from medicines, hormones, and genetically modified DNA of the body as well as poisoning from the cowmilk. In many cases its calcium will float in your blood without being properly used. Raw milk from healthy animals fed on healthy natural grasslands is far better, if you need milk in your daily food mix.

What happened in history of men is that we are completely disconnected from the function of the mouth. The love for nature and food and the pleasure of nurturing our body with healthy food is far away for many people.

When we understand and respect the system and our body, we will increase a healthy, shiny and fresh mouth. The chewing of the food with the right amount of moisture for mixing from our glands and preparing the mixture for our stomach and pancreas in our conscious behaviour will increase the happiness and beauty of our body and life. When everything is in balance again many diseases will disappear. And it is not a big effort when we do it out of love for ourselves, unless we have issues about loving and respecting ourselves...

Unhealthy teeth and cavities are causing imbalances and diseases in the body. It all starts with the mouth; it is the starting point of our daily live in eating and talking and partly breathing.

The energy (frequencies) of words influence the energy in our mouth. There is a saying when somebody is expressing dirty or negative words: "go rinse your mouth". This is so true, because if you don't, you swallow that energy with water and food into your body which will have certain consequences. You can speak of "instant karma" in this case.

The worrying thing is that a lot of this was already known in 1800 and dr. Price did research in the 1920's of last century. You can say that not so many people were educated in that time. But the educated dentists and doctors could have informed each other and the patients. But the reverse effect occurred: The more education and schools in last 100 years the worse the teeth became and the more cavities. This is because the basic principles of living here on earth are not taught on schools or at home.

The colour and brightness of the teeth gives also indications about health or mental state. For exampleyellow coloured teeth might indicate some issues with the liver environment.

Channel on emotional eating

What is the relation between emotion and digesting?

Good morning Hans, interesting question you ask. Digesting food is digesting environment. But since you do not eat from your environment, you also digest from your planet, so it is more active and sometimes more passive (because passive energy). It is a complex situation, but let's go to the basics.

You eat to stay alive in your prospect/perception. That's ok, but what you eat is who you are or how you feel. So, it is correct that you are going to eat, in this case, because of the feeling/emotions

*to digest this, because you do not allow the feeling. You want it to
stop/go away fast. The issue is to separate emotional eating from
feeding yourself. Yes, it works, but the guilt feeling afterwards
brings you down. The exercise is to go in the emotion-feeling
and live it "alive" (in the moment). So, take your time, when
you are alone and don't want to share or are not able to share the
emotion. The unrest from the emotion field is not dangerous, but
it is a habit from the past and you know that! Yes, it is confusing,
because of some reverse spinning energies, but live it and in
the future, this will be the habit. Set the triggers on the eating,
processing habits and reverse that habit vortex, so it will vanish
away. The food tastes, you mentioned, are triggers for you. You
look for food from the past. When you set those triggers and the
food is not there, you look for replacements, but those are not good
enough, so you keep going on... Release the original trigger tastes
in combination with that emotional-feeling. You are a sensitive
person and many food-related emotional memories are in your
system.*

Channel on healthy food

*What is right food for healthy teeth? Food is a subject for many of
you. You wonder if you are doing it right. It is your intention that
you are doing it with, not a mental choice. You will feel what is
right, not programming and scheduling your food. Inform yourself
with "your" right sources and feel what is good for you and your
system. Do not obstipate on this subject. Be yourself and not be
afraid. Lose habits of eating and try again and again and again.
Channel on specific subjects for your personal health. It has to do
with your origin, living area and in which life stage you are. Do
not force, your body knows, listen and do what feels good.*

*For tooth issues do not point at food specific, but you need to be
healthy in basic. Adjust what suits you in your environment right
now.*

Learn from your environment, taste and experience.

Humans change and so do food habits. Do not underestimate your feelings and power in this. Taste, select and combine. Make wise selections in the now, not history. The food you needed for your earlier experiences does not exist anymore. There is no right or wrong.

We are your earth-family who will support you in what to do with water and food. Change your water when needed for your system. Water is from the gods of the universe, combined with stars energy. You are the stars; you drink the stars. You eat the earth; you are the earth. The sun powers you and makes you smile. Enjoy your day.

How do teeth work?

Teeth are alive

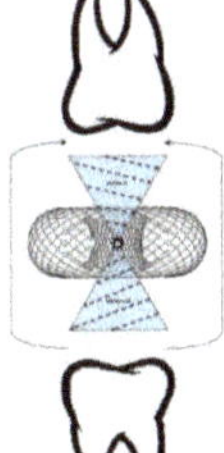

Teeth are living beings with consciousness! What earlier already was found about hormones, saliva, tooth protection and the vortex between upper and lower teeth comes to a new level now. The saliva which is protecting, cleaning and informing the teeth is not coming from outside the tooth, but from inside. With healthy teeth and healthy connections to other body parts and systems, the vortex influence on the tooth is having the tooth fluid coming out. If there are unhealthy circumstances the vortex may reverse and sucking the mouth fluids, including unhealthy, unbalanced components directly into the tooth, the blood, nervous system, etc. This can cause many problems on short and long term. And when the unstable situation continues for longer period, it will go fast.

Just like we humans like to be in friendly and save environment, the teeth, gums and jaws like that too. Why do we protect little children, animals, etc. and not our own teeth and body?

So, our task is to give the teeth this environment where they can grow, shine, interact with you and represent you. Just like hands, face, feet and other body parts, the mouth shows who and what you are. So, shining from inside can also been seen through your smile and healthy teeth, gums and jaws. It is not about a nice organized row of teeth, but the total energy from that area what other people observe. And in communication the biggest part is subconscious exchange.

In fact, we have 32 children in our mouth, who like to be loved, nurtured and fed. They all have their emotions and can act like people doing in a group. They play, fight, dance and love and they can be strong, shy, lonely, etc.

Teeth show emotions by color, position and direction, pain or can even be damaged when the emotion stays a long time.

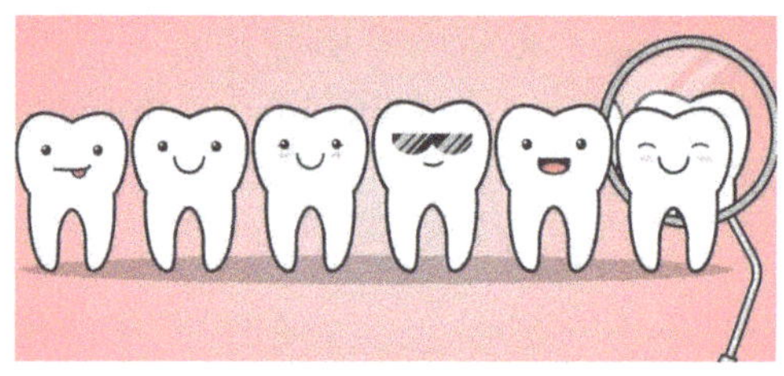

This is also the reason why suddenly one tooth starts to feel hurt or even get sick or damaged. If all the teeth are a part of you, the signal of that tooth is a signal from a part of you. In the mirror you can see many aspects of you, also in the teeth.

Channel on healing the vortices

Can I heal the vortex of the teeth?

What you ask is intriguing. What shall we do with that? The Vortex is the result of what is going on/playing in a subject or object. There is no right or wrong, there is just spinning from our side of the view. You observed on teeth and in the past on chakra's a double vortex and in case of unbalance one spinning seems stronger than the other one, so it is attracting stronger.
Yes, interesting question that everything should be in balance…but then there is no flow, no direction, no life! So that's the reason you observe a direction. The key question is if you "force" direction

from outside if then the attraction in your life will change and the old issue disappears? Yes and no. Yes, you can change it and it works, but "client" can shift it back, when nothing changes in his/ her life, just like any other healing. So, you can experiment with that and see what works. You can start with the teeth drawing and Pendle, but later you will observe it and change it directly. Make client aware and issues can come up or choices in her/his life will popup after changing it, so client must be aware of that. So, it is combi healing and that's strong. In general, you will learn more on reversed spinning and how to adjust the right speed. Yes, fillings have to be removed first until you understand to heal/ recover/regrow damaged teeth directly. So, enjoy it.

A vortex is pulling and not pushing. Pushing is forcing and pulling gives the opportunity to fill that space with new energy. That energy will spin in that system in the right direction and vibration. Pushing is releasing of "old" energies. The direction is interesting and you will find out when objects/energy spin right and when left on your planet. So, start and I will download your visibility on vortices, so you will notice them in seeing/feeling the "speed" and direction. Enjoy.

Yes, your thoughts were ahead, but that's trust and what is time...?

Lol

Where to start (my question) Top-down and front-back or reverse?

Look at the influences, first the ones that influence others and yes top-down is best, but again...what is time and sequence of it...

Addition: Is it possible to do vortex teeth healing on implants?

Yes, it is possible but be careful to first learn that specific tooth that it is ok and will not be pushed out. Better is to test the direction and speed and see the influences and work on issue healing. Later we help you in working on replacing fillings with the original material and recover the tooth in a healthy one. Enjoy your sunny day.

The teeth are alive research

That teeth are alive is scientific proven and known, only not teached or shared with the rest of the world. This should be teached at schools. When this info about the working of the teeth is integrated in our daily life it becomes natural to take care of it. The reality is that corporations imprint different information in society and dentist and that info is now the "reality" for the society. The change of this belief system can change when you start to change yours and act on it.

How does that fluid system work?

Dentin and enamel are living tissues, normally fed with blood. In all the teeth we find many odontoblasts. See below pictures.

Odontoblasts form the dentine, a collagen-based mineralized tissue, through secretion of its collagenous and noncollagenous organic matrix components and by control the mineralization process. A conspicuous cell process arises from the cell body of odontoblasts and penetrates into the mineralized dentine. After dentinogenesis, odontoblasts deposit new layers of dentine throughout life and might also form a type of reactionary/ reparative dentine in response to dental caries and other external factors may affect teeth.

The odontoblasts are kind of pumpsystem for the fluid, containing many minerals. On the outer side, in the mouth, the fluid protects the teeth and rebuild the tooth, when damaged.

In this case the odontoblasts filter from blood what is needed for dentin tissue to keep it alive and healthy.

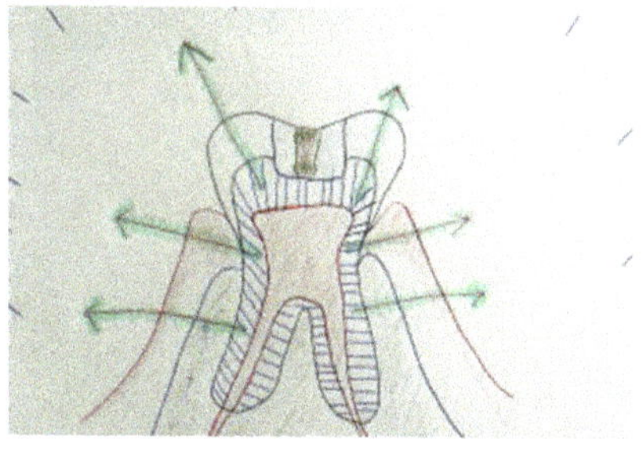

So, if blood is not in balance, the teeth show that too in colors and energy.

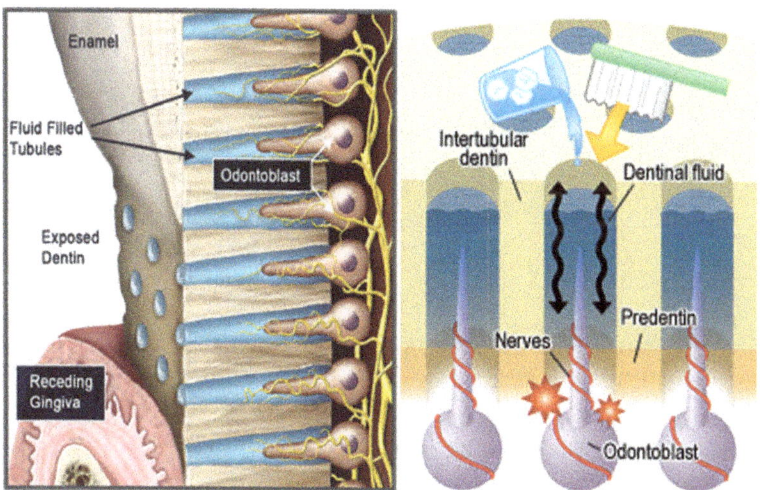

The odontoblasts are kind of pumpsystem. So, if enamel shows cracks, the pressure difference is lower and fluid flow increases for protection. The odontoblasts feed also the

minerals for enamel mineralization when needed for repair
or (re)grow.

And they also regulate the PH required in every situation.
The PH of Dental Fluid mirrors the PH of the blood. So,
everything connects with everything. Healthy blood helps
healthy teeth!

The pump systems can be influenced too. This means
lower capacity or even reversed working, like I showed
earlier. This means that, in this reversed case, the fluid
from the mouth goes into the teeth. Imagine that you are
using toothpaste, which has a label: "do not swallow". This
chemical goes in the tooth, when the tooth is unhealthy at
that moment. This risk is also strong when we are eating
artificial/chemical sugars. In fact, it can be disturbed by
anything in the mouth, which the body does not recognize.
Now we are back at the important subject: good nutrition!

Hormones, Glands and teeth

The fluids in the teeth and mouth and the digestion
components and organ activation is coordinated by the
body systems. An important system for this is coming
from the glands. The big coordinator for the mouth is the
Hypothalamus.

The Hypothalamus reacts on the food coming into the
mouth and the Parotid gland produces less or more fluids
for protecting the teeth and preparing the digesting process
in the organs in line for digesting.

Sugars and carbohydrate diets reverse the protection flow
of the fluids through the teeth mainly. Maybe we can say
in general: "natural foods will be supported and the rest

can damage the fluid protection and without protection it damages the teeth" I that case the teeth are attaked from 2 sides. The bad nutrition destabilizes the body inside and the teeth inside and also on the outside of the teeth.

It is all about attention, intention and focus, see influences in picture below:

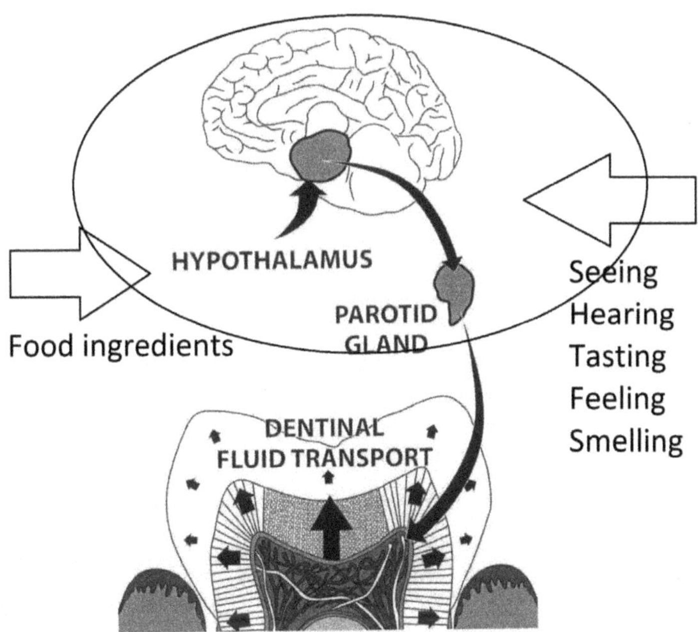

Diagram representing the human Hypotalamus-Parotid gland Endocrine Axia (HPEA)

With the right attention, intention and focus the vortices around the teeth are directed in your way, for you and you are a healthy, living being.

Example about focus: when you are eating in a restaurant

you are focussed on the ingredients, tastes and smells in
the right atmosphere. So, the experience of a restaurant is
in many cases more related to the food en environment.
When people are eating at home, many people are doing
that in front of TV, PC, Mobile, Newspaper or have other
distractions. The digestion fluids and hormons will be
influenced by focus on these impulses and information.
You eat what you see, hear, so...that "information" you eat
is going into the body and those energies with information
is digested and will be used in your life. Be aware how
the systems work and how it original was meant to be in a
natural way.

The gland system is very important for the teeth
health. It starts with the interaction of pituitary gland
and hypothalamus. The pituitary gland stimulates the
parathyroids which controls the calcium balance in the
system. See more about this below. The Hypothalamus
is very important in stimulating the parotid glands for
digestion enzyme production and stabilizing the mouth
bacterial culture.

Also, the 5 Tonsils (see pic) have important functions in
keeping teeth and mouth healthy.

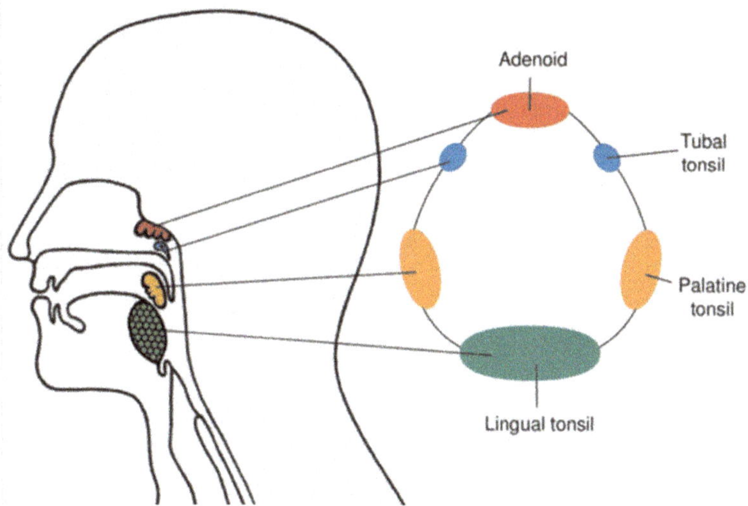

This is ring of glands and tonsils is called "W-ring".

The hormone system balance is important for healthy teeth and healthy body function. One of the aspects is the balance of the Vitamine A and D (cod liver oil, fermented) which stimulates the balance of the Calcium, phosphorus and K2 vitamin/mineral in the systems.

The hormone system and Glands immediately react on different kinds of food. The natural "cleansing" of the teeth is always in function. Although with certain foods, like sucrose diet, stops the fluid and in that case the effect is double worse: bad food in body and no natural cleaning! This is why the chemical sugars are so bad for the body and teeth. The body system has problems with detecting these unnatural components.

Tooth repairs and fillings can influence the system, because of the "disturbed natural exchange". The root canal treatments for example and the poisoning of that process also creates problems in Tonsils and hypothalamus which creates unbalances in the natural working system. The body is so complex and has internal and external so many connections and influences that only holistic approach can identify what is going on. And on that level issues can be changed and corrected to its natural state.

In the past dentists thought Fluor was good for preventing and recovering caries. But in fact, green tea works better and Fluor is dangerous for the brain, glands and the rest of the body.

Vitamin K2 is the most natural way to organize the best teeth health. It works on Hypothalamus and indirect on Parotid gland for making teeth fluid for keeping the environment of the mouth and teeth clean. K2 is natural available in raw milk and fermented cheese and some vegetables. Or you can look for K2 supplement, which your body can accept and use.

Calcium, Hypothalamus and absorption

The hypothalamus controls the hormones for the right absorbing of the calcium components into the body and the right distribution. Cow milk adds components which disturbs this process. The use of animal milk is originated from society believes and genetics on a created "dependency" on animal milk. If your body needs cowmilk, use the more natural form. Raw milk from natural cows has a better balance for our systems than processed milk from chemical manipulated, GMO cows. Component balance is destroyed in the process of heating and filtering and intentions and disbelieves. The genetic manipulation, medicines, hormons and bad food have changed a natural cow into a chemical factory cow. But some people try to work with more natural cows in more natural environment. This good intention works also in the love for the animals and a healthier milk.

The hormone imbalances disturb also the enlightment, connections with pineal, thyroid and pituitary glands. The addictions we created in our systems sabotage our believes and feelings, so we think we are doing right. Be careful with testing on this and the body feelings. Ask others to help you in the first steps. The addictions are based on wormholes, implants and believes in your fields and systems. This is more "technical stuff" for energetic healers.

Parathyroid hormone regulates the body's calcium levels

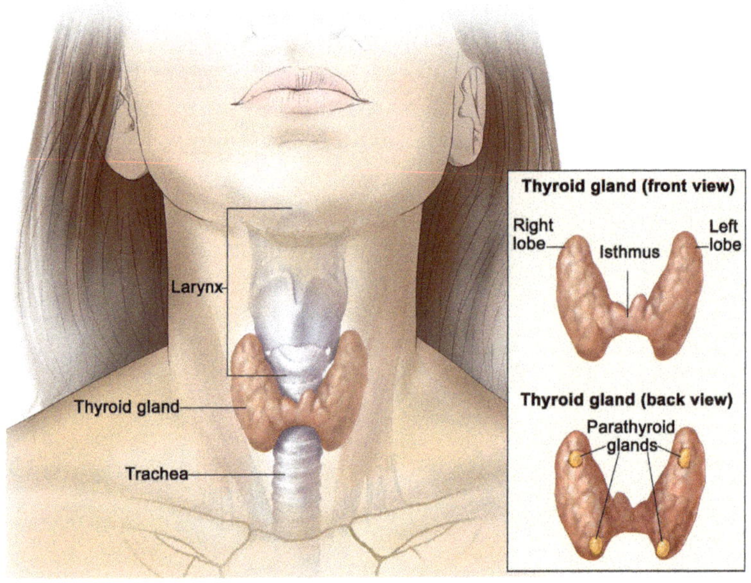

Anatomy of the Parathyroid Glands

The four parathyroids are typically found on the back side of the thyroid. They're about the size and shape of a grain of rice.

The parathyroid essentially helps the nervous and muscular systems function properly. Calcium is the primary element that causes muscles to contract and calcium levels are very important to the normal conduction of electrical currents along nerves.

Although the parathyroids are very close to the thyroid gland anatomically, they have no related function, according to science. The thyroid gland regulates the body's metabolism, while parathyroid glands regulate calcium levels and have no effect on metabolism.

Parathyroid Hormone

Parathyroid hormone (PTH) has a very powerful influence on the cells of your bones by causing them to release their calcium into the bloodstream.

- PTH regulates how much calcium is absorbed from your diet, how much calcium is excreted by your kidneys, and how much calcium is stored in your bones.

- We store many pounds of calcium in our bones, and it is readily available to the rest of the body at the request of the parathyroid glands.

- PTH increases the formation of active vitamin D, and it is active vitamin D that increases intestinal calcium and phosphorus absorption.

Diseases and Disorders of the Parathyroid

When the parathyroid releases too much or too little PTH, it adversely affects your body in a variety of ways. Below are common diseases and disorders associated with the parathyroid glands:

- **Hyperparathyroidism:** The most common disease of parathyroid glands is hyperparathyroidism, which is characterized by excess PTH hormone, regardless of calcium levels. In other words, the parathyroid glands continue to make large amounts of PTH even when the calcium level is normal, and they should not be making the hormone at all.

- **Hypoparathyroidism:** Hypoparathyroidism is the combination of symptoms due to inadequate parathyroid hormone production. This leads to decreased blood levels of calcium (hypocalcemia) and increased levels of blood phosphorus (hyperphosphatemia). This is a rare condition and most commonly occurs because of damage or removal of parathyroid glands during parathyroid or thyroid surgery.

- **Osteoporosis:** When one of the parathyroid glands is overactive, it releases too much PTH hormone. This causes your bones to release calcium constantly into the blood stream. Without enough calcium in your bones, they lose their density and hardness. Osteoporosis is characterized by this loss of calcium and bone density.

The parathyroid glands have a single responsibility — regulating calcium levels. The glands are important members of endocrine system, but they are also integral to the proper functioning of the nervous and muscular systems.

Channel about parathyroids

What are Parathyroids and why 4?

I'm educated by many lives on earth as healer, medicin woman (and man) and was teached about your creation as humans and development. Hormons and fluid stuff is my specialism.

I'm in your feeling female with Elfin energy, but in fact I'm not. Happy to get you informed about this subject. Hormones are material and non material to start with. It is as usual double (yes, I'm working with your brain words for establishing a better connection to you). The double is of course for the human experience, but in fact it is not. The most important, as you discovered already, is the energy, resonance and light colors and frequency combinations. Hormone stuff, in material, you can read in medical articles.

Calcium is the crystalline manifestation of your building material, like the pyramids in the middle of a desert with sand. (note from me: she means in an environment without enough Calcium). Can Calcium be in the body without calcium food? Yeeaah you know it can. It is coming from outside (or inside) from moving consciousness fields ordering itself in the right resonance for manifestation(materialisation) for your body and calcium is binding(chemical) in resonance to the right other components to be transported in the body, so it can shift its combination depending on the location in the body.

All 4 of the Parathyroids have different functions on this and their "task". But they are coordinating in that "place" (thyroid) in the body because of the growing (body growth) balance between up(head) and down(body). It is also working with the Thyroid on growing balance based on DNA, food, country region, etc. So, the food is scanned by lips, W-ring, Parathyroids, lungs and diaphragm. With all that info the body knows what to do with food. Calcium is from many different outside sources and like blood it carries "DNA" information from its origin, like mother or cows. So, calcium can be left unbounded in the blood, because it is rejected by your body of its origin. It is kind of poisoning frequency. You can transform it, clean it or remove it. Calcium is catalytic and can be split/grow/divide itself in more, like cells, to be used in the body. The right Calcium is from natural plants, but also from from fish or meat, if natural, healthy was the state of the being. Also, water and air is a source for multiplying calcium.

The ring of 4 has nothing to do with the 4 heart chambers, because they work simultaneously (and the heart serial...) for the balanced info. It is combining info to the centre point and they each can take over each other tasks if necessary. Local stem cells can create extra cells to activate that. Calcium is important for many functions in the body. In the jaws is Calcium stored for teeth growth and if teeth regrow or repair itself the jaw calcium will be rebalanced to the right level. Amalgam is reducing calcium in jaws, because of the electrical tension. So, Amalgam can cause more cavities in your teeth. The Parathyroids are stimulated by the Hypothalamus and informed by the Pineal gland (DNA info) and other sources outside the body fields and sources in universe.

The salivary gland secretes saliva

Here some information from the science and research about this subject.

(Secretion is the movement of material from one point to another chemicals, or a secreted chemical substance from a cell or gland.)

The salivary gland secretes saliva. The salivary gland secretes saliva that helps us chew and swallow the food we eat. The pancreas secretes digestive juices that enable our bodies to break down the fat, protein, and carbohydrates in the food. Secretions like these are important in countless activities that keep our bodies running day and night. A study published today in the journal Science Signaling uncovers a previously mysterious process that makes these secretions possible.

At the heart of the new study is calcium, which is present in all of our cells and is a gatekeeper of sorts: an increase in calcium in our cells opens up "gates" or "channels" that are required for the production and secretion of fluids like saliva. If calcium doesn't increase inside cells the gates won't open, a problem that occurs in diseases like Sjögren's syndrome. Sjögren's patients experience dry mouth due to a lack of saliva and have difficulty chewing, swallowing, and speaking, which severely hampers quality of life.

For the past 15 years David I. Yule, Ph.D., professor in the department of Pharmacology and Physiology at the University of Rochester School of Medicine and Dentistry has studied calcium's role in Sjögren's and other disorders in which calcium and secretions are disrupted, like acute pancreatitis. In the new study he answers an important question that has stumped scientists for years: what does it take for a particularly important calcium channel to open and start these processes?

Scientists have known that the presence of a protein called the IP3 receptor is necessary to increase calcium and generate channels in many, if not all, cells. But, the IP3 receptor is complex: one channel is created from four identical units in the IP3 receptor, and it was not known how many of the individual units had to be engaged for the channel to work.

Using advanced molecular engineering and gene editing techniques driven by Kamil Alzayady, Ph.D., research assistant professor in the Yule lab, the team discovered that, without exception, all four parts must be activated (turned on) for calcium to increase in a cell and start processes like fluid secretion. Yule believes this feature ensures that the calcium channel only opens under strict conditions that result in secretions, avoiding harmful events that would occur if the channel could open more easily. (Paradoxically, too much calcium is also bad and can lead to processes that kill cells. So, it is no surprise that cells keep tight control over calcium levels).

The Hypothalamus and the Pituitary Gland

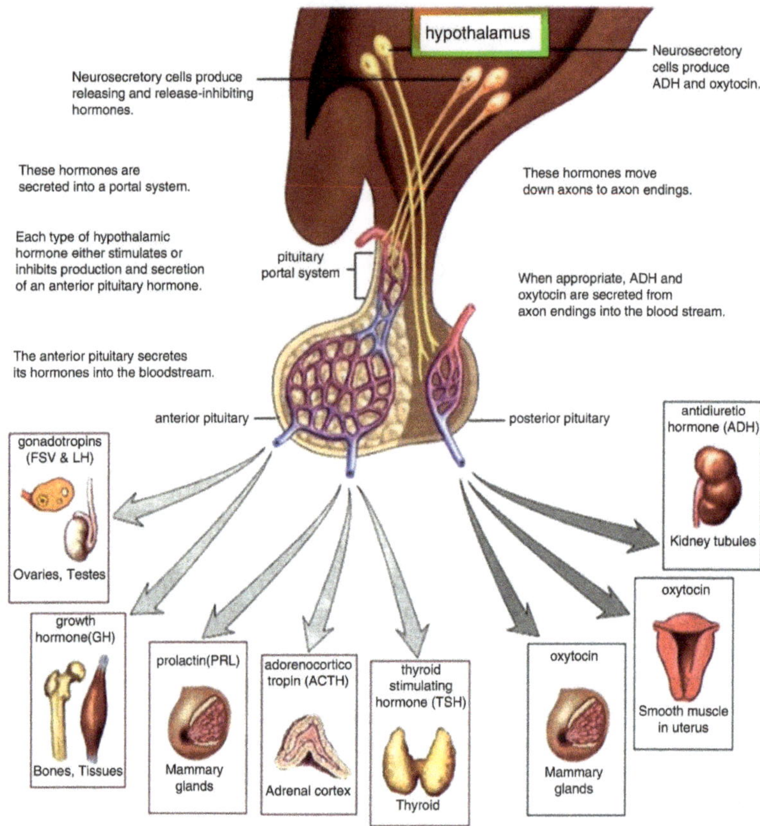

The hypothalamus is the region of the brain that controls hormone release, and is thus part of the neuroendocrine system. The pituitary gland is closely allied with the hypothalamus, both functionally and physically. Some hypothalamic neurons project directly to the neural lobe of the pituitary. Others project to the median eminence, where they connect with blood vessels that supply the pituitary. In either case, the hypothalamic neurons influence cells of the pituitary, either upregulating or downregulating their activity. Hormones secreted from the pituitary in turn influence neurons throughout the brain (including the hypothalamus), and endocrine glands located in other parts of the body such as the adrenal, pineal, thyroid, parathyroid, thymus, heart, stomach, duodenum, pancreas, testes, ovaries, and placenta.

The Hypothalamus is also the stimulating gland for the thyroid gland.

What is relation between teeth and our life?

The next part explains the relation between teeth issues and problems/diseases with organs. There are repeating correlations between body parts and teeth. We can origin that maybe to meridian energy lines. We have earlier discussed the many system interacting between teeth and the rest of the body. And with the body we move in life and the body memory stores and uses that memory and "programming" again in other experiences in life. If I jump to the short connection between teeth and life, this makes sense? So, life is connected to the teeth and teeth are connected to your life experiences. What can we do with this? We listen to the teeth and watch them and most important: feel them... all of them!

If we look at the mouth we can see and dedicate many signs and symbolic to the structure, like following picture shows. The terms spirit, mind, etc. can be different or have a different feeling, depending of the information and experiences you received in life. I only use it to make it a little clear for the brain.

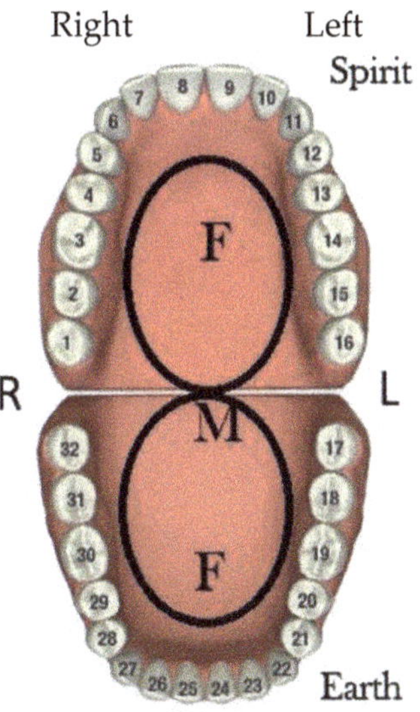

If we see the mouth as female and the tongue as male, we can see following picture and energy flowing. So, one of the aspects is the balancing between male and female aspects and energies in the human system.

The upper jaw is symbolic for spiritual and mind connections and the under jaw for connection with the earth and life.

The upper jaw is connected to the skull bones and the under jaw with under body, like arms, hips, legs and feet. These connections we saw in the earlier pictures.

So, we can make connections between teeth in upper jaw and the spiritual development and systems (like chakra's and aura layers) and the teeth in under jaw with more earth connected functions in body, like walking, moving and acting in life.

So, the mouth integrates both aspects in one system, spirit (and mind) and body in balance. The connections from the teeth to the organs and the tongue to the organs is an interesting aspect of the mouth. What we see, if we tune in, that in fact every organ is connected to every organ, see the example picture below.

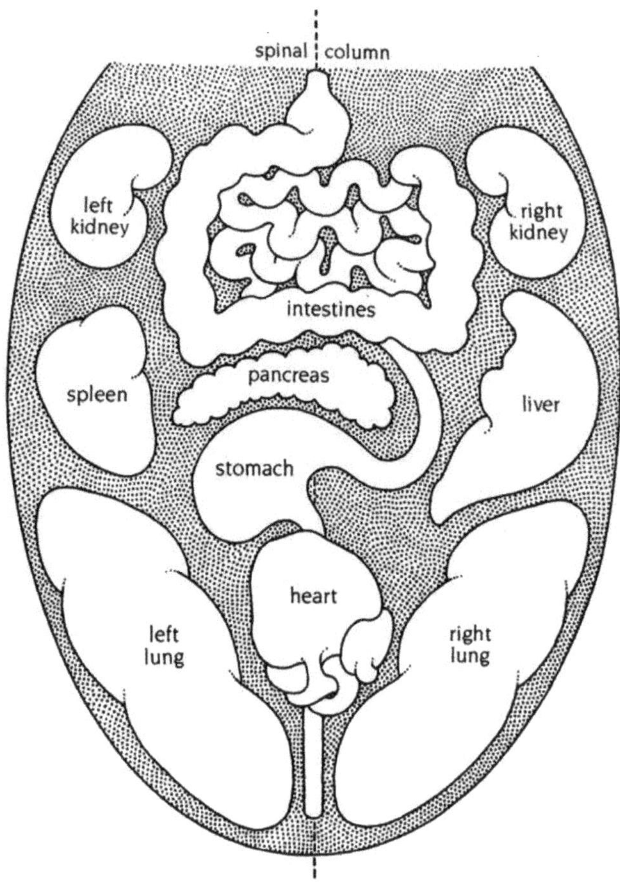

So, as explained earlier, there is no one way direction, like many medical people and dentist think or know. It is more complex and we need always to find out what is the issue which causes the unbalance in the different parts of the body.

The teeth are connected to the chakras from personal self

and higher self. The chakra's have both energies of male/
female or right/left as vortex running (or turning). So,
depending on the issues one of the vortices maybe more
dominant in the chakra and not in balance.

The front of the body is connected to the future and the back
to the past.

There are also aura layers involved, but that is not 1 on 1
connected like the info I just mentioned.

The meridians are the (ley)lines connecting higher energies
with body parts.

The teeth are very good signal receivers and indicators.
The connections from the teeth and the meaning of the
unbalance can tell a lot about what is going on in a person,
even if the person is not yet (complete) aware what is
"playing behind the scenes".

Jaws interpretation

These mentioned meanings are general interpretations.
We always have to look at the complete picture of the
mouth, teeth and jaws in combination what is going on in
the life of the person. I mention below some other possible
"connections/interpretations".

If upper jaw is bigger than lower jaw then the person is
more in wishing and thinking then doing and manifesting.
If lower jaw is inside upper jaw, the person is not strong
expressing and doing. Keeps everything hidden for outside
world.

If upper jaw is small, there are issues with authority from
outside, like parents or other entities. If lower jaw is big, the

person is more acting from instinct then thinking about the action.

When the left side or the right side makes the lower jaw out of horizontal balance then there is an unbalance between the imagination and manifestation on male or female subjects. This is in many cases the result of unbalanced crawling as child where the brain parts are interacting and joining the actions.

If front teeth are not touching and there is a gap (up and below), that means a trauma with fright and or amazement(astonishment). It has also to do with trauma wish to be more physical connected to one of the parents. If they used left thumb it is more mother (or inner female) oriented and with right thumb more father (or inner male energy) oriented. The thumb is symbolic for personality in this case.

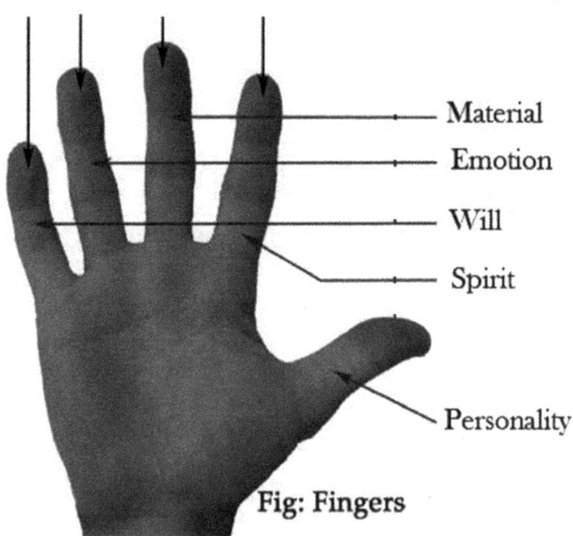

Fig: Fingers

If people are chewing on the right (80%!) that has consequences for inner balance and how the approach life.

If there is overbyte, the mental is strong and first thinking
and thinking...and then doing under control of thinking. If
the gap (from front to back) between upper front teeth and
lower front teeth is big, then there is a lot of space between
thinking and doing.

Underbyte is the opposite.

Little kids, like to put a finger in their mouth, pushing on
upper front teeth in more or less strong force. This is all
symbolic for their lives.

Another meaning is giving and receiving. Upper jaw and lip
are giving and lower jaw and lip are for receiving.

Upper Jaw is desire, wishes.

Lower Jaw is realizing, manifesting.

Chewing is mixing creations with manifestations for the
process of digesting.

If the tooth is directed inward it is self oriented, outward
directed is directed on others. Introvert and extravert is also
connected to this. Teeth moving and/or pointing more to
the front is future oriented (or fear from the past). And of
course, everything is a mirror so the last point we can also
use on all the other orientations of the teeth.

Symbolic of teeth

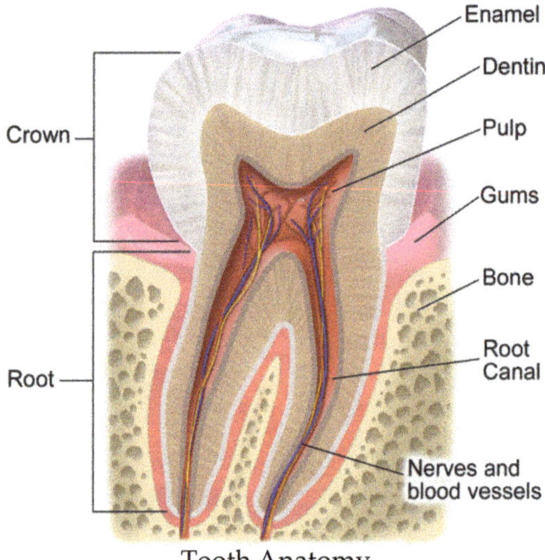

Tooth Anatomy

The Enamel is the visible part of the tooth, how you show yourself on that energy. It is also your protection on that energy, how to set your borders in life.

The Dentin is the form of the tooth, the model. It represents life inside you, your form, model.

The Pulp is your health. How is the feeding of the tooth, the energy for feeding the Dentin and enamel, the feeding of your shining light?

The root is how that energy is fixed, grounded in your life. Also feeling comfortable, welcome, feeling protected, fed, loved.

Position in jaw. Is the tooth directed to your inside world or to the outside world? What is the position to the teeth surrounding that tooth?

The jaw is the fundament of your life. How have you created the basics of your life you wanted and feel good about.

Channel about tooth construction

Symbolic of tooth construction

Tooth Enamel is symbolic for strength, power, shining energy by its position and pointing direction. It is masculine energy with female soft protection, yes masculine protected by female energy, ironic, not?

The part (dentin) between the life, health and vitality inside the tooth is filtering that energy and life, showing in Enamel. If the pulp is dead the enamel is dead.

The root is in the womb of the jaw, so the masculine enamel is pointing out of the female womb, like vagina.

This is also protecting the tooth. The root point is in the soft womb to make it more comfortable while chewing. That's better than fixed directly. That's also better when changing teeth during youth.

What is symbolic for missing a tooth, so you have had no birth to that energy and interaction/sharing with others (teeth).

When a tooth is removed it is "killed" or stopped. Just like other removed parts in the body, it will "kill" some experience or just gives you an extra experience.

When a tooth is horizontal (in jaw) like wisdom teeth sometimes do, it is the opposite of co-working, it is solo working, doing what it (= you) want with no line, no guidance. So, out of line in strong way. This is in lot of cases family or ancestor or society energy. It gives you a challenge to realign, to grow up.

Broken teeth are something you really do not want; you break it without "killing" it.

Mouth coherence with 32 children? Hahaha, good luck! No balance, no compassion and harmony in life. Doing what you want in line with your spirit.

About vertical vortex, we share with you the abundance when vortex is in optimal speed, direction and strength (size of vortex). You can test on that too. Strength is giving something (tooth meaning) space to live, to grow, to BE!

So Thats's all.

Have fun.

Gums

What is the "behind cause" and symbolic of gum diseases or problems? In a lot of cases it is disbalance between calcium and phosphorus. The shortage of vitamin B12 can be a problem source too.

What is the understanding for the behaviour of the gums?

Gums are symbolic the whomb of your teeth, the comfortable chair the teeth are sitting in. So, are you/feel supported in a warm, comfortable and lovely environment? Are you feeding yourself (besides the food) with comfort, energy, love, joy and relaxation?

But the proper food is also very important. Are you taking care of yourself and your body?

It has also to do with pushing yourself too much, going over your limits, borders, etc. This is also resulting in the body reaction that the sympathic(nerve) system will be too long in action. The sympathic and parasympathic movements should alternate and not stay a long time in one over activation.

The Calcium and phosphorus balance can be disturbed by sugar. If your Parasympathic nervous system is dominant it needs to be triggered by Calcium or sugar.

Your system always looks for solutions for you, so if you are addicted to speed the nervous system, the system will ask for sugars.

Another problem for the gums is aggressive use of teeth, too much pressure on the gums. This is caused by hard chewing, long term pressure and unnatural long forces like for example jumping with skeleton, for example in sports.

All supplements needed for (re)balancing, must be the right ones for the body to accept them and use them in the right way in the right place of the body. See earlier in this book about testing yourself on these subjects and supplements and how to do that.

Teeth symbolic from front to rear

The backside of the mouth has to do with soul (teeth 8) and the front side with the now, your appearance in life. Everything in between can be the filters, blockings, etc. in your life. It is your way and experience in life. How you express yourself, interact with others and of course how you interact with yourself. How are you "eating/biting" through life. Are you processing(chewing) life in awareness, or bite and swallow fast? Are you aware of your chewing and tasting when you eat?

Channel about Wisdom teeth

Why 4 wisdom teeth and what is connection to the heart?

Hello goodmorning wisdom "freak". You wanted to know about wisdom teeth? What is wisdom? Is that knowledge? Inner feeling? It is inner truth, you know what is right or wrong in your duality, it is what suits best for you in that moment. Is it innerguiding? Yes, kind of. The four teeth are the four directions left-right and above-below. Left-right can be direction but also the meanings you already know. Above-below is the greater view or the smaller part, universe-earth or spirit-material (body).

So yes, in fact it is part of heart connection, but also feeling, so it is more complicated. It is your guiding in life to feel (know) that you are right in that moment. So, is external (universe/spirit) knowledge wisdom? No, you only know/feel that the connection info is right for you. So, what happens if the wisdom teeth are not there? Are you stupid then? No! The only thing is that you have issues on that. You don't want clear guidance or in your case you "disturbed" guidance shows you what happens in life. Do you need them? No not with your present food consumption. Interesting new aspect... "evolution" or adaption of human body to new circumstances in life, food and environment.

So, there are many things connected to those 4. Are they connected to the 4 heart chambers? Yes and no! The heart chambers have each a passing of blood and air(yes!) connected to 4 "stages" of the soul. So, the guidance from the heart for you here on earth is kind of guidance, but not the 4 directions from wisdom teeth. The 4 chambers have to do with your movement as human on earth in full integration in body. If you are fully in balance, your heart is in balance in all 4 stages, 2 arms, 2 legs, oeps...now you understand and so... yes heart has also so above so below. Upper chambers arms and lower chambers legs connections. So why heart attack in left arm. It depends on issue of the attack, but in your life era/period it is of feeling, feminine aspect on your doing, that is left arm. Is that upper left wisdom tooth? No, both left upper and lower wisdom teeth.

Is it wise hahaha, to regrow wisdom teeth, if they are removed or not present? No, just balance the issues and put it back in energy with all connections of blood, nerves, lymfe, meridians, etc. and aura layers! That's all.

So, lots of new info today. Have a lovely day.

What about cleaning?

Toothpaste

Test for yourself which toothpaste is ok for you. Forget all regular chemical toothpastes from the big corporations in the supermarket, whatever they claim. Use f.e. clay type toothpaste or other natural combinations of ingredients. If it is not advised to swallow it by the corporations, it is of course unhealthy. There are many recopies on internet to make your own natural toothpaste.

Definitively through away all stuff with fluor! It is chemical poison in the way they produce this technical fluor.

As you fully believe that teeth are selfhealing, cleaning and protecting you can consider only to floss and brush with water. Floss is now also possible with waterfloss systems. But only do this if you are convinced and in full trust to do it and take your responsibility for it. Consider the natural way the body works, but on the other side be conscious about your type of food intake patterns during the day. If you allow yourself to take food, which might not so good for teeth, do some extra cleaning afterwards.

Cleaning and food

Teeth are natural protected, but the way we live and eat makes it necessary to clean them. The most important parts to clean is between the teeth. Special when you eat snacks, like bread, crackers, cookies, etc. This food leaves little parts between the teeth. And as mentioned before, the components, like sugar can cause unbalance in the mouth and damage to the teeth.

Cleaning teeth is sensitive subject in this society and the only person responsible for any consequence is yourself. Even the dental "care" industry has legally covered this any advice in their terms and conditions, when you do "business" with them.

Observe your teeth daily, feel what the different kinds of food do with your teeth and adapt your behaviours and food. Everything is about being conscious in your life about your habits, choices and focus. It is not about being "bad" or have to punish yourself, but be aware and choose.

Oilpulling

Here a description from internet, what it is. Find your own way in this process.

Oil pulling is the practice of swishing or holding oils from plants in the mouth for long periods of time to produce health benefits. It is an ancient folk remedy that has been researched, and while not all of the claims of oil pulling enthusiasts are true, oil pulling does have its uses.

Enthusiasts of oil pulling, also called Kavala Graha or Gandusha, claim that toxins and bacteria in the body build up in the mouth and that swishing or holding oil in the mouth for a prolonged amount of time will draw out these impurities or wash them from the mouth. Once the swishing is complete, the oil is spit out into a sink or trash basket.

"The whole purpose of oil pulling is to get rid of the oil-soluble toxins in the body," said Puneet Nanda, creator of GuruNanda

Pulling Oil and founder of Dr. Fresh Oral Care Line.

Some popular oils used in oil pulling are sunflower, coconut, sesame, olive and palm. While coconut is one of the most popular pulling oils, it becomes a solid below 75 degrees Fahrenheit (23.9 Celsius), creating a chunk that is hard to swish around in the mouth. "But when blended in correct proportion with sesame and sunflower oil for the purpose of achieving a doshic balance and a more thorough detox, the mixture will not harden," said Nanda.

In the Ayurvedic health care tradition, doshas are bodily energies that determine a person's prakruti, or one's physical, physiologic and mental character and disease vulnerability. Factors such as stress, unhealthy diet, weather and strained relationships can all influence the balance that exists between a person's doshas. These unbalanced energies in turn leave individuals more susceptible to disease, according to the University of Maryland Medical Center.

Oil pulling is also used for dental purposes. Many claims that it strengthens gums, whitens teeth and eliminates plaque. Others use it as a treatment for TMJ, an ailment of the jaw.

A more extreme use for oil pulling is the treatment of disease. Some say that oil pulling cures cancer and other diseases by pulling toxins out of the body. In fact, oil pulling is cited as a cure for 30 different diseases.

You have to feel how long and often you do this. My experience is to do this in the beginning a few times longer (15-20 min) and later for maintenance only 5-10 min. But many people have many different opinions about this. I created my own oil for this with ingredients for healthy gums and teeth. There is a lot of suggestions available on internet.

Is there a connection between Teeth and diseases?

As we have seen, there are many connections from mouth to other organs and body parts. There are also many processes going on in the mouth for protecting, cleaning all what is going on there. Imbalances in the mouth can cause imbalances in other parts of the body.

I have listed some recent literature and research info which seems to be in interaction with our mouth. The below subjects are just for illustration what science thinks and how things are connected in the body.

Pancreatic cancer risk

From a research it was found that the connection to pancreas is connected to 2 bacteria:

- Porphyromonas gingivalis
- Aggregatibacter actinomycetemcomitans

These 2 are in the mouth connected to poor oral health (self love) and inflammations.

Gingipains are key factors in tissue damage symptoms of periodontitis, which results from the degradation of matrix metalloproteins, collagen, and fibronectin. Degradation of these substrates interferes with interactions between host cells and the extracellular matrix, therefore impeding wound healing and causing destruction of periodontal tissues. Rgp is responsible for eliciting the host inflammatory response via the $p38\alpha$ MAPK transduction pathway. This response likely contributes to

the inflammatory nature of periodontitis and is involved in
tissue and bone destruction

From statistics came that these bacteria had a strong relation
to Pancreas cancer risk.

Parallel is there also the connection to heart problems with
these bacteria.

Rheumatoid Arthritis

*In some cases, gum-disease causing oral bacteria may set off a
cascade of events that leads to the autoimmune form of arthritis.*

*The Porphyromonas gingivalis bacteria are also connected to
Rheumatic arthritis.*

*The most accurate marker for RA-found in the blood of 76% of
the RA patients- is anticitrullinated protein antibodies (ACPA's)
These antibodies target citrullinatedproteins that are xepressed by
immune cells such as neutrophils. This can cause joint-destroying
inflammation.*

This all is in strong relation to gum-disease.

*Calcium is required for citrullination. In the study, Aa produced
a toxin that punched holes in neutrophil membranes, allowing
calcium to flow into the cells in greater-than normal amounts. The
excess calcium amplified citrullination, resulting in the patterns of
hypercitrullination seen in RA.*

Note:

Has to do with too much or wrong Calcium or Calcium
poisoning from cow milk. It is in many cases a genetic issue.
This can be solved by looking in your issues behind this

process and in family behaviour.

Has to do with guilt, sorrow, resentment programs in the micro plasma. They think they have to fight for everything and do not want to change or move.

Cognitive functions and tooth loss

From studies it was shown that loss of cognitive functions a relation between the number of lost teeth and the risk. In this research the group characteristics were taken into consideration, like smoking, diabetes, etc., but without strokes or dementia.

Table 1. Baseline characteristics of subjects who underwent dental examination

Characteristics	Dental examination n = 438 (67%)	No dental examination n = 212 (33%)	P value
Mean age ± SD (yr)	63 ± 7.9	62.5 ± 8.0	0.07
Gender, No (%)			0.24
Male	123 (28.0)	69 (32.5)	
Female	315 (72.0)	143 (67.5)	
Education, No (%)			0.15
≤ 6 yr	213 (48.6)	116 (54.7)	
≥ 7 yr	225 (64.2)	96 (45.3)	
Hypertension, No (%)			0.15
No	157 (35.8)	64 (30.1)	
Yes	281 (64.2)	148 (69.9)	
Diabetes mellitus, No (%)			0.08
No	338 (77)	150 (70)	
Yes	100 (23)	62 (30)	
Current smoking, No (%)			0.01
No	388 (88.6)	172 (81.1)	
Yes	50 (11.4)	40 (18.9)	
Hyperlipidemia, No (%)			0.38
No	288 (65.9)	147 (69.3)	
Yes	149 (34.1)	65 (30.7)	

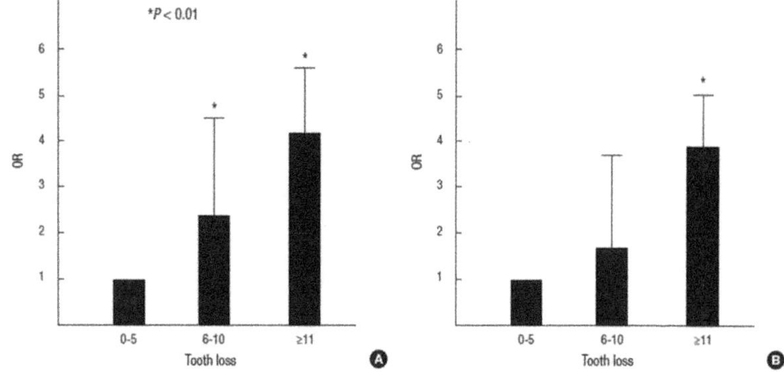

Cardiovascular disease

Conclusion from Indian report. It is now clear from the epidemiologic studies that a potential link does exist between PD and CVD. Oral healthcare professionals can identify patients who are unaware of their risk of developing serious complications as a result of CVD and who are in need of medical intervention.

But also in the united states many statistics are published. There is a big connection between root canal treatments and heart attacks in these statistics.

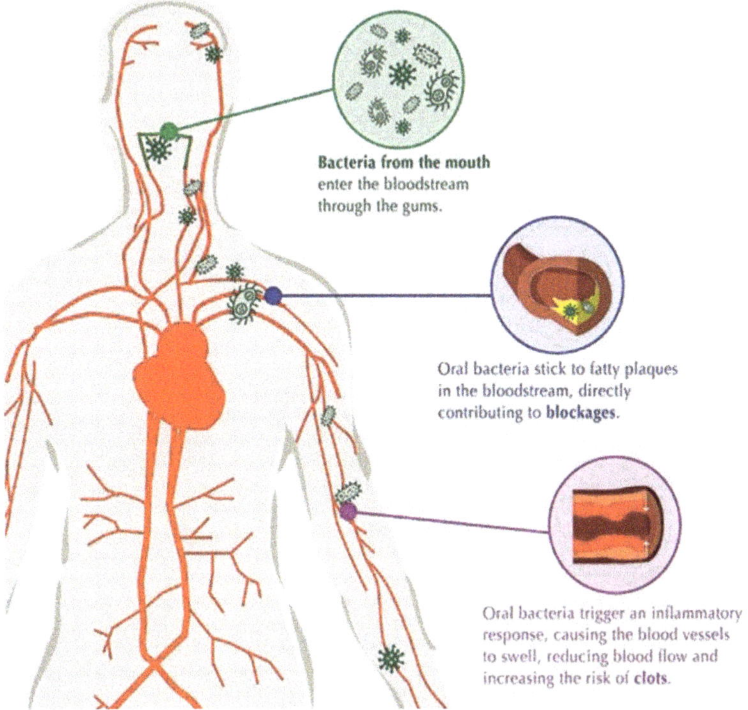

Note:

Like in this picture, science finds bacteria in different places and makes the connection, but hardly ever they turn it around like "is the root cause in the heart or in gums". In many minds is the heart the victim of the process. The holistic way is to look at the bigger picture. What you eat, do in live, interactions with others, history of family, past/ parallel live connections, etc.

The question is if the tooth/gum problem is causing the health problem or reverse. Or is it maybe all the same based on the same belief issues in the body field system?

Do I need fillings?

If a tooth needs to be filled according to your personal feeling (the dentist can advice you) you can choose from many materials. Nowadays Amalgam is out of the question because of the poisonous ingredients. Many dentists are replacing these fillings for new materials.

If you observe your cavities, look at the cause. The first thing with cavities is to look at your nutrition, cleaning and check (with healer) if there are (emotional or trauma) issues in your life connected to that specific tooth.

Another thing with fillings is the look of the dental industry on teeth. For them, teeth are a kind of rock you can fill with materials, like an old house. But earlier we have seen that teeth are alive and breathing through the materials. So, if you close a part of the tooth with impenetrable materials, something is not in balance there anymore. The healthy and protecting fluids are blocked in those filled parts of the tooth. The important thing is to recognize the signals of the teeth long before the big cavity is there to show you that something is really wrong.

Amalgam

A lot of filled teeth are treated in the past with Amalgam filling material, containing mercury and other stuff. The poisoning material is entering many organs in the body, some meridians, brains, lymphe system and the pineal gland.

The most dangerous parts are Mercury, Silver, Zinc, Copper, Tin and the glue. This must be removed from the body by healing techniques or herbs or other ways.

It looks like it is possible to clean the components with herbs, oils and other natural techniques, however it still occurs in places where life issues are stored. Even when cleaning with energy it remains there. After solving the issues, where it was connected to, the component energy is removed. If we look it that way the Amalgam had a function to show us our issues in life, but in another place than the teeth.

When removing Amalgam fillings by a dentist, here are some tips:

- Choose the right dentist for you who has at least good experience with removing and is not placing new Amalgam fillings at all.

- The dentist should use the Swedish protocol. The use of rubber dam around the tooth is controversial, so feel if you need that. And discuss with the dentist what is the best for you.

- Test how many fillings per treatment is possible for your health. Remove all fillings in one session can be too much for the body.

- Test the sequence of the removing fillings. If Amalgam is combined with gold, do that one first. If the gold part remains in the tooth, the poison has to be removed from the gold by healing.

- Use extra vitamins and minerals to help the body with removing poisonous components like C, B6, B1, Zinc, Magnesium, E, Selenium, Bromelain, etc.

Safe filling materials

Are there safe filling materials? That is a personal matter, so you have to check what your body can accept. Choose also the dentist where you feel comfortable with to carry out the filling.

All fillings have some positive and negative properties. F.e. gold looks save, but pure gold is too soft and needs to be mixed with other materials. So, the best is to investigate yourself and let your body decide what feels the best in combination with the choice of dentist, who can do it. Holistic, biological dentists are more open to suggestions from their clients.

Root Canal treatment

One of the books I read was referring about long time investigations of root canal treatments. They explained the complexity and the toxic results and diseases this can result in. A big investigation was already documented in 1923, but was completely ignored by the dental organizations, who keep saying that it was completely save. The same story about amalgam fillings. In recent years the amalgam story is changing, because a lot of dentist are open now to remove the toxic and electrical and electromagnetic poisoning fillings.

The writers explained the poisoning of the body specific on the root canal treatments. It is very detailed what they found out in the visible and measureable area. Can you imagine what happens on energetic and consciousness level in the body system. There is a relation between root canal treatment and heart attacks in their statistics.

Dentist are conditioned (by education) to save teeth from extraction. Certainly, one reason is that it is a reasonable goal to preserve functional teeth. However, the rest of the body should not have to pay the price. Another reason is that root canal procedures are high-profit dental treatments. In addition, root canal procedures result in performing more crowns and bridges. These procedures also generate large profits in a dental practice, since fewer teeth are extracted and can be sources of repeated various procedures for years to come. So again: follow the money and you know what's going on.

I am not supporting to remove all damaged teeth, but observe what is going on in dentistry. Dentists are the first observers of problems and should be able to help clients in preventing, teaching, healing etc. which can be profitable for dentist and client.

There are many diseases and psychic issues related to tooth problems and specific to root canal treatments and the poisoning from that.

One of the poisoning effects is reducing the enzyme CPK (Creatine PhosphoKinase) necessary for ATP balance in the body parts.

The best thing to do is prevent it. Observe and "listen" to the teeth and nourish them and take care of yourself.

Bracelets

Another interesting article I read was about bracelets. There was described how the fixing of the teeth in a nice order can be faster and better accomplished with less pain with sounds and specific body movements. This has to do with body connections to and from the teeth. Moshe Feldenkrais did many investigations and treatments with body movements.

Bracelets can cause reshapes of the head and TMJ problems! See further in this book about TMJ. Also, other tooth problems can cause hurts in neck, ears, eyes because of all kinds of tensions.

As mentioned before the jaws are connected in many ways with the body, also by bones and muscles. There is a relation between the use of bracelets and changing the form of the head.

Why are the teeth not always nice organized in the jaws and why are they sometimes start to turn or walk? This question can only be answered by the tooth itself. Observing with logical can give you some info too, like why is the tooth directed inside or outside or hiding beyond the neighbour teeth?

Why change my teeth in colour?

As mentioned before, teeth are good signal instruments to show you (in mirror) what is going on. If you look regularly to your teeth, you can see that during the day (food, drinks) or emotional periods the colour of the teeth change.

We explained before that the fluid flow and the possible reversed operation in the tooth can cause effects, which you can see in colour. In science is also proved that when you put a coloured fluid on your (mouth) glands, it appears fast at your teeth. The circumstances and balance in your mouth is shown in the colour of your teeth.

So, food, drinks, emotions, environmental influences can change the colour of your teeth.

When you can look almost into the core of your teeth, because they are very thin on the outside, it means you need to change food, minerals and maybe the way you live. Start with the check of Calcium, phosphorus and K2.

Can I get new teeth?

Sometimes we read this kind of messages:

Tooth began to grow in the month of 104-year-old woman
(03.02.2001 Source: Pravda.Ru).

*A 104-year-old patient of Drozhonosk District Hospital, the
republic of Tatarstan, Russia, surprised doctors by saying that
new tooth began to grow in her month. It is a unique case,
Tatarstan Health Ministry reported. A few cases of adults' tooth
renewal were mentioned in the Guinness Book. But it has never
happened to a person, who is more than 100 years old. Three teeth
are simultaneously growing in the month of Maria Vasilieva. She
is glad about it. "Now I'll be able to eat spice-cakes", the long-
liver says. Local dentists observe this infrequent phenomenon.
The woman lives alone. Her husband and children died long ago.
She runs the house, keeps poultry and a kitchen garden, keeps
an eye on TV and radio news. In this thinly populated district of
Tatarstan there are 8 persons over one hundred years old. But only
Maria Vasilieva has new tooth.*

Other stories from internet to show that the way of thinking
is changing:

*After all, when a tooth is broken or falls out, it's not like when
you cut your nails or shave your beard -- that ain't growing back.
Well, actually, that might not be the case for long, as there are
not one, but two teams who've set their sights on taking down the
denture industry by regrowing your very own teeth right inside
your very own mouth-hole.*

*First, there's a team from the University of Alberta in Canada
(where hockey-related tooth loss strikes virtually every male before
age 15) who say they've managed to regrow broken teeth by using
ultrasound emitters. Seriously, they just point sound waves at*

your teeth and they grow back. The procedure worked so well on rabbits that the scientists figured, screw it, why not scale up the difficulty and try it out on an animal whose entire diet isn't just cabbage and water? So they tested a variant of their ultrasound method on humans and found that it worked, even when the root itself was damaged. The system consists of a "miniaturized system-on-a-chip" that constantly barrages the root of your tooth with good tooth vibes as you wear it inside your mouth, and in no time ("no time" meaning "about a year") you're right back to popping beer bottle caps with your pearly whites.

More recently, a bunch of researchers from Columbia University and Nova Southeastern University in Florida have said they can regrow teeth using dental stem cells. When a patient loses a tooth, the docs simply plop some dental stem cells into a tooth-shaped scaffold and wait for the stem cells to work their magic. The patients can grow the new tooth either inside their own mouth or outside the body, but either way, within nine weeks they've got themselves a shiny new food masher. And no, the stem cells being used for this procedure don't come from embryos. Instead, they're collected from discarded teeth or other "dental waste," which we sincerely hope isn't as gross as it sounds (but probably is).

On internet we find more and more articles about people who discover third generation tooth in their mouth. Sometimes this happens by surprise, in other cases it happens by meditation, focus and manifestation techniques.

In all literature the main thing is focus on the root of the teeth. This is where the stem cells will be activated for regrowing a new tooth or reconstructing a broken tooth. Healing cavities by focus also happens. There are now also chemical products for healing and reactivating the healing of enamel cavities available. In literature we find that there should be genes responsible for third (or later) series of new teeth. The gene seems to be activated in a certain time period, so then the issue is to reactivate that gene again when you want a new one. Meditation techniques show results by different type of focussing techniques. So, there is no general effective technique yet available. See below a basic meditation and find your way in this.

Stem cells

There is a lot of research going on in science with stem cells. Below picture is the most natural way. But still carried out outside the body in laboratory. Recent they start to test on animals, but if that is the right way?

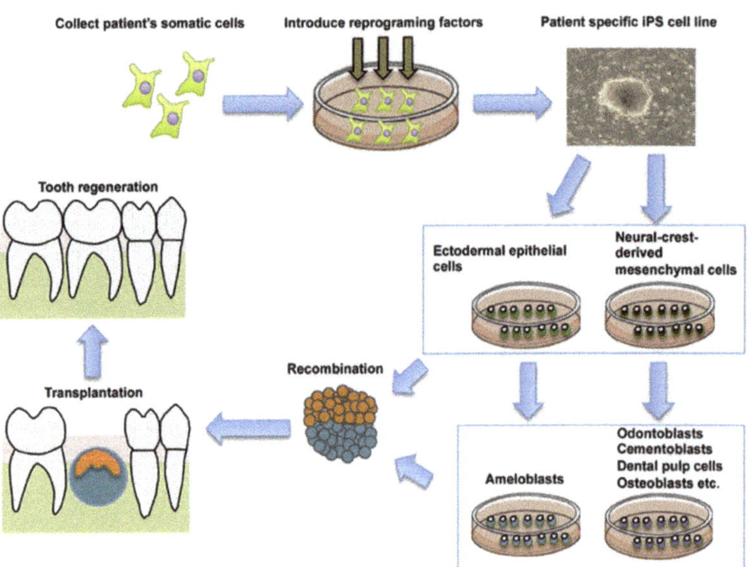

It should be possible to instruct stem cells inside the body to do it. More investigation is necessary. In my workshops for healers I share a technique, which I received by channel. What I discovered myself is that hidden thoughts behind the mental reason why we want to have new teeth can block the process. So, the first step is to clear that way and look at the hidden programs and expectations.

Channel on stem cells

What about stem cells?

Stem cells are arbitrary phenomenon. It is used in human Medicin world, but in fact every cell is a kind of stem cell. It is only the control of it which makes it specific for that purpose. Medical will understand in future, but it is not the time yet, just like with free energy. Stem cells are controlled by the Hypothalamus and programmed by pineal gland and supported by pituitary and local glands for the local use of the stem cells. Stem cells are in that case Mastercells determined for a specific goal, like creating new organs, new tissue and change of the functions in that area. So, stem cells are personal and kept being alive outside a body but still connected and controlled by that body in a certain way. They can be influenced by hormone fluids locally. So, a mixed environment can exist in that way. It is not meant to be in that way. Your researchers will find that out later. Stem cells for teeth growth have to be in the right environment and is controlled by DNA. Wild teeth cells are normally not possible. It has to be done carefully, but is possible.

Yes, we can help you later when you understand more about the working of the body and teeth. We will guide you before with info. First the complex material of connections, because that is important for the regrow of new teeth and disconnecting with "old" teeth. The removed ones remain in established function but outside the body. Isn't that remarkable? So, study this complex material and we will come back. Enjoy this exciting ride of teeth, be careful and take care.

We are always here.

Regenerating teeth meditation example

It has been proven that we can regrow our teeth by meditation and changing our believe system. Viewing regrowing teeth animations will help to in your belief that it is possible.

1. Concentrate on the root of the tooth in the jaw, which can be regenerated, even if there is a part or dead tooth located.

2. Imagine that there are stem cells (approx 12-24) on that spot on the root. Imagine that these stem cells are activated to grow a new tooth, just like seeds of plants in the soil.

3. Imagine and feel that the tooth is growing from those stem cells, like a little plant is growing.

4. See and feel that the little new tooth is pushing out the rest of the old tooth and is coming to the surface.

5. Enjoy the feeling and view of that new tooth in that place of your jaw.

6. Keep repeating this every day.

TMJ and TMD...or TMJD, what is TMJ?

TMJ stands for *Temporo Mandibular Joint*, which is the hinge joint that connects the lower jaw to the temporal bone of the skull, which is immediately in front of the ear on each side of your head. The joints are flexible, which allows the jaw to move smoothly up and down, and side to side. This smooth motion allows you to talk, chew and yawn. Muscles attached to and surrounding the jaw joint control the position and movement of the jaw. Commonly, disorders of the TMJ are incorrectly called TMJ, but should be called TMJD: Temporo Mandibular Joint Disorders/Disfunctions. But in literature it is most called TMD.

What is TMD?

TMD, which stands for Temporo Mandibular joint Disfunction, happens as a result of problems with the jaw, jaw joint and surrounding facial muscles that control chewing and moving the jaw. The causes of TMD are not always clear, but dentists believe that symptoms arise from problems with the muscles of the jaw or with the parts of the joint itself.

Injury to your jaw, the TMJ or muscles of the head and neck (you might be experiencing neck pain or headaches in Atlanta), can cause TMD. Some other causes of TMD might be:

- Grinding or clenching your teeth, placing pressure on the TMJ.

- Dislocation of the soft cushion or disc between the ball and socket.

- Presence of osteoarthritis or rheumatoid arthritis in the TMJ.

- Stress that causes you to tighten your facial and jaw muscles or clench your teeth.

In this chapter I only mention the short subjects about TMJ. The TMJ is very important, but there is a lot of literature and help available in books and online. Below I show what I found important from literature and my experiences in my practise. To solve it we need to reprogram the body behaviour by repeating the new way of moving and resting the body. From childhood we learned to walk, move and eat, so to change these patterns it can take some time. Be patient and enjoy it.

**NORMAL TMJ
MOUTH OPEN**

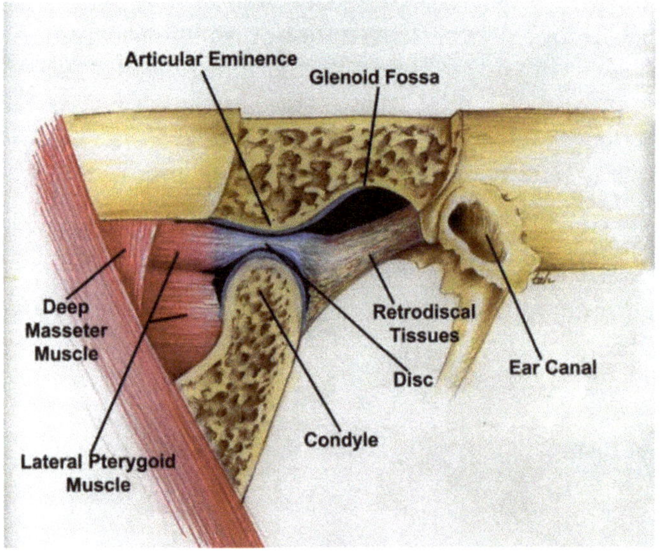

ABNORMAL TMJ
ANTERIORLY DISPLACED DISC

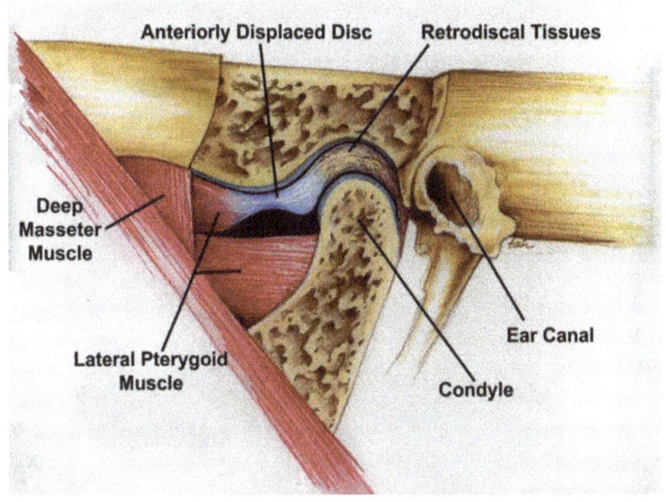

ANTERIORLY DISPLACED DISC
WITH CHANGES IN SHAPE AND OTHER
DEGENERATIVE CHANGES

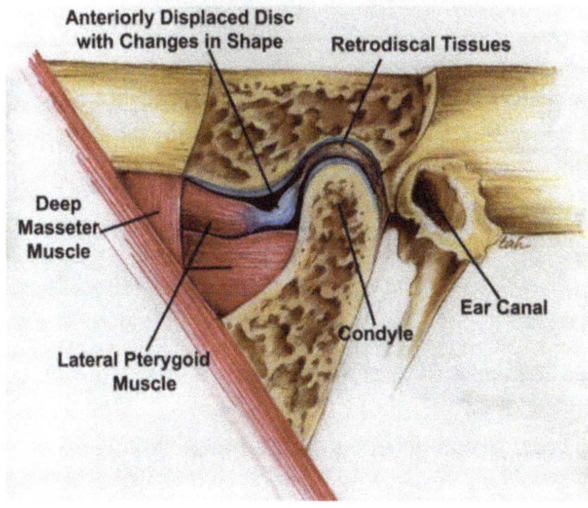

What are the symptoms and causes of TMD?

If you suffer from TMD, you might experience severe pain and discomfort in the craniofacial region that is either temporary or lasts for many years. Some of the common symptoms of TMD include:

- Facial pain
- Limited ability to open mouth
- Jaw gets "stuck" or "locks"
- Tired feeling in the face
- Difficulty chewing or a sudden uncomfortable bite
- Swelling on the side of the face

Some other common symptoms of TMD might include toothaches, neck aches, dizziness, earaches, hearing problems and headaches in Atlanta.

On internet you find good videos explaining what happens with the TMJ. One of the reasons the TMJ get in trouble is because of jaw movements. The upper jaw exists of 2 parts connected in the middle by a flexible connection. Due to several causes the upper jaw can push upward and give a smaller face. This can cause nose and breathing problems, because the maxilla blocks the open air space of the nose, the nasal passageway.

This TMD is caused by movement of the jaw. Why is the jaw moving? Here is one reason:

There is a general "rule": Teeth dominate, muscles and joints accommodate, so it stands to reason that the jaw joint will accommodate as well as it can.

Mouth breathing causes stress on TMJ by pulling the lower jaw backwards. See further the part about breathing and

TMJ.

Even tooth extraction can cause TMD. Mainly removing wisdom teeth cause many TMJ problems. This has to do with movement of teeth, tongue, etc. Causing disbalance in the system, causing the TMJ displacing, etc. Dr. Mike Mew did much research in this area.

When teeth are out of position the lower jaw can shift to the left or right, causing a asymmetric lower face and imbalance of both TMJ's.

TMD has the effect (or interaction!) with the neck and causes FHP (Forward Head Posture).

So, to cure the TMD is first be aware and correct lower jaw and at the same time correct your posture, like with Moshe Feldenkrais practices. These are anyway good for posture, breathing and overall health.

All of above-mentioned dispositions can be related to any tooth problem. Like expressed before, it is very important to have the complete view of body, movements and energy fields to start with the correction of the TMD.

What to check?

If one of these general problems occur, we need to see the overall picture of what is happening. Back to the root of all and ask yourself following questions:

- What is body posture?
- What is neck posture?
- What is head posture?
- How do I swallow?
- How do I breathe?

If not ok, work on it by practises your posture and
movements of the parts.

- What is size of upper jaw?
- What is size of lower jaw?
- What is the position of lower jaw?

These tensions can be released by focussing, belief work and
orthodontists

Mouth breading? Very important to work on issues and in
daily life and why it is happening.

When you have TMD and want to correct it, you have to
start at the beginning, the posture, breathing and be aware
how you move.

It is just like a building, you need a good foundation, floors,
roofs and interior design. So, we need to rebuild from the
floor and step by step reprogramming the body posture and
movement in life.

What can be done about TMD?

Many possibilities and solutions, there is no line in that. In
medical world are many therapies available:

- Surgery
- Placing part of rib behind to block the backwards
movement
- Fysiotherapy
- In between bracelets, splint
- Hypnosis
- And many, many others

What can you do yourself?

Posture focus.

We are coming back to the important experience here on earth, the body! We have a body and learned how to use it and move with it. But are we using it in a comfortable way? To feel and understand the comfortable positions of skeleton and muscles we have to start at the beginning. Standing, sitting and sleeping are much used positions in life. Standing is for humans more complex then animals with 4 legs.

- Balance your feet, so both legs are equally charged. Check why it is comfortable in different position. Where in the body feels more comfortable in unequal position?

- Feet in the normal forward direction. Check also why it makes comfortable to do different. Where in the body feels more comfortable in unequal position?

- Switch the charge per leg on regular basis, body is made for movement.

- Head in upright position looking horizontal.

- Shoulders little backwards, so your thumbs are facing forward.

- When walking, the arms move relaxed in opposite direction of the legs.

Sitting in a chair the same. Feet flat on the floor and straight back. What makes you comfortable to sit different? Try and feel other positions.

- Arms relaxed and supported.

- Try to get the TV, book or computer higher with the top close to eyebrow level.

- Move every 20-30 minutes and walk to activate the body.

Sleeping positions are on the side or on the back. If you sleep on the stomach, something is creating that, like digestion problems, fears, or...On stomach laying forces the neck in uncomfortable positions.

Make sure the pillow supports the neck in both mentioned situations. You can use other pillows to support legs or arms, if you need or want that.

When we go to the head posture there are very important basics. Mouth closed. Lips together, tongue on roof of the mouth, teeth not touching and jaw muscles and mind relaxed. Avoid bracing, clenching and grinding. Drugs can influence these last phenomena too. If your tongue is not naturally "fixed" on the roof of the mouth and you focus on changing, it can be confusing in the beginning. After a while it happens automatically when you combine the lips, mouth and tongue positions.

Channel about Tongue position

Tongue info

The knowledge of the tongue is deep rooted in life (deep rooted inside you). There are many sayings in life, like "talking with split tongue", "sharp tongue", etc. This is all true and possible to express. Receiving energies from different tongues. So, you see different energies, different receiving, different emotions. Yes, the tongue is male and female for its expressions and energies towards yourself and others. The construction of the tongue in relation to the mouth is more male. It is always more (or less), never only male or female.

The tongue has many organs connected (like every other part of the body), so the tongue speaks from your body, your experience, your life. This is sensed by others. Yes, speaking is also possible to read (analyse/interpretation) like on feet, teeth, face, eyes, etc.

All is one and one is all. So, you attract people on your speaking in combination with sound, feeling. So, it is…YOU! Your expression attracts others. You cannot hide. You can change, improve, learn by being open, open in receiving and open in sending.

Yes, the tongue is a strong muscle, but the sending energy doesn't have to be like that. If we speak through humans, we can use voice, tongue, etc. To get the right vibration out for that moment. Is that you or is that us, what they receive in that case? Both, it is a mix!

So now more internally spoken your tongue doesn't need to rest, it can work all day, just like horses don't sleep much. Sleeping is other subject Hans. So, the tongue is laying on top or on bottom of the mouth, or moving around. Preferred when you sleep, and no brain thinking, the tongue can help you and your energy by laying on top. This is also for safety by the swallowing. This is natural automatic, let is happen.

Touching with tongue your teeth can have different reasons. It can contact for transferring energy or controlling if everything in the mouth is alright. The teeth and tongue are very sensitive in that. If the tongue is doing that out of discomfort, there is discomfort, unrest in your system. Do you need to control everything? Interesting fact is the position in the backside of the mouth. The tongue can close and open that portal there for all kinds of reasons, it is also a gatekeeper for what is going in or out.

The roughness on the tongue is caused by little "sensors" which can be normal, hyper or even irritated. This is also about you.

Colors of the tongue are also signals about your state, your health.

The tongue is at the position of TMJ and yes in direction of inner hearing and inner aligning. So, you can express from your inner self by letting that energy move your tongue from backside or sharp from mental, then the form of the tongue will change.

Yes, they say tip of the tongue is heart point, but is not for healing. The heart energy comes from within, so if the tip signals heart, it is in most cases lack of the heart energy flowing from the backside of the tongue.

Breathing and TMJ

Many problems in the body start with wrong breathing. The breathing can subconsciously change by many reasons in our growing up in life. When it starts early in life it is strong programmed in the body and needs more attention and focus to change it back in the natural way. One off the problems is mouth breathing. When you look around many people breath through the mouth for long times and you can see that they do it subconscious.

Breathing has direct influence on your being. It is making connection with the soul.

Northwestern Medicine scientists have discovered for the first time that the rhythm of breathing creates electrical activity in the human brain that enhances emotional judgments and memory recall. These effects on behavior depend critically on whether you inhale or exhale and whether you breathe through the nose or mouth.

In the study, individuals were able to identify a fearful face more quickly if they encountered the face when breathing in compared to breathing out. Individuals also were more likely to remember an object if they encountered it on the inhaled breath than the exhaled one. The effect disappeared if breathing was through the mouth. "One of the major findings in this study is that there is a dramatic difference in brain activity in the amygdala and hippocampus during inhalation compared with exhalation,"

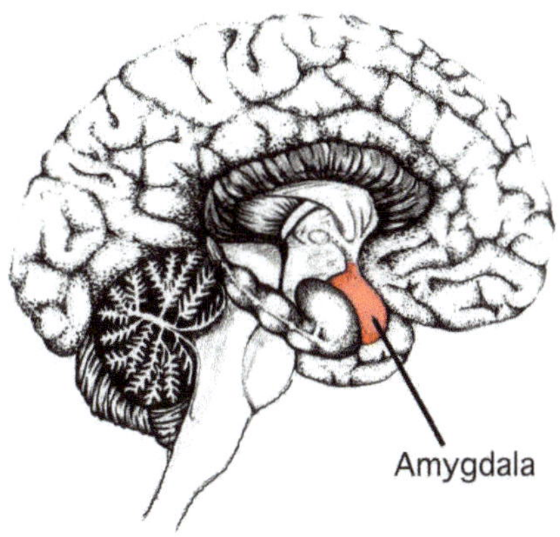

Breathing through mouth connects more to the mental brain.

There has been much research on mouth breathing, TMJ, tonsils, etc. The sequential order can differ but there is a connection between the physical parts around the mouth. One effect of mouth breathing can be a disorder on the upper jaw, which will not make a round form, but more reversed V-shape. This causes a problem for the air intake by the nose. The other problem can be an infection or milk poisoning on the Tonsils by nose or by air pollution by breathing through the mouth. This can result in taking away your tonsils, like doctors did in the past with young children. Tonsils are important for our health, food processing and other functions.

Breathing through nose is important, but breathing by diaphragm is also essential for our existence. Diaphragm can be stuck, locked or block in other ways that breathing and attention is going to the lower part of the body and the lower chakras. Good information you can find on the website of Heartmath institute and GCI, Global coherence initiative.

Breathing is life, so do it in the right way. Belly breathing by Diaphragm is the standard way and is possible to learn the body to do that. Sometimes you need the higher ribcage breathing or in extreme circumstances breathing through the mouth is necessary. How are you breathing? Sometimes people open their mouth when they listen with strong focus as if the words go through the mouth to the ears. Those are learned reflexes of the body which can be changed.

Muscles and TMJ

The muscles are very important for the movement and location of the lower jaw. Without the muscles we cannot speak, sing, eat, swallow and breath(mouth).

Many TMJ problems are caused by muscle movement. The jaw-muscles there are so strong, they can press up to 80 kg! This can also cause pains in jaw, neck and head. Because we move a lot with the mouth muscles. Also passing emotions can be stored there and even can lock, stress or frustrate the lower jaw movement. These frustrated muscles can keep things in a circle:

Pain – tension – circulation (muscle fluids, food, waste) reduction – movement is restricted – muscle inflamed – pain

In a lot of cases these muscle stress has to do with anger, frustration, unspoken issues, internal fights, sleep fights, etc.

Tight muscles can hurt jaws and teeth and even damage the teeth. Also, tight jaws during the night can cause headache and neck pains in the morning.

Practice in sensing (feeling) the muscles and relax them and relax the jaw. Do this all day and you will sense the lower jaw going back in a more relaxed natural position. There are many muscles connected to the face and jaws and are connected to the central facial nerve.

The muscle pains will show (feel) themselves in many places on your head. Besides solving the programs, believes, emotions, feelings, pains, grief, etc. also restoring the relaxed state by relaxing massages and acupressure will help to regain the original relaxed state. In many cases we already kept that stress for a long time and the cells remember the position, tension, etc.

This is all about being aware and change your habits and life.

Do you suffer from any of the following?

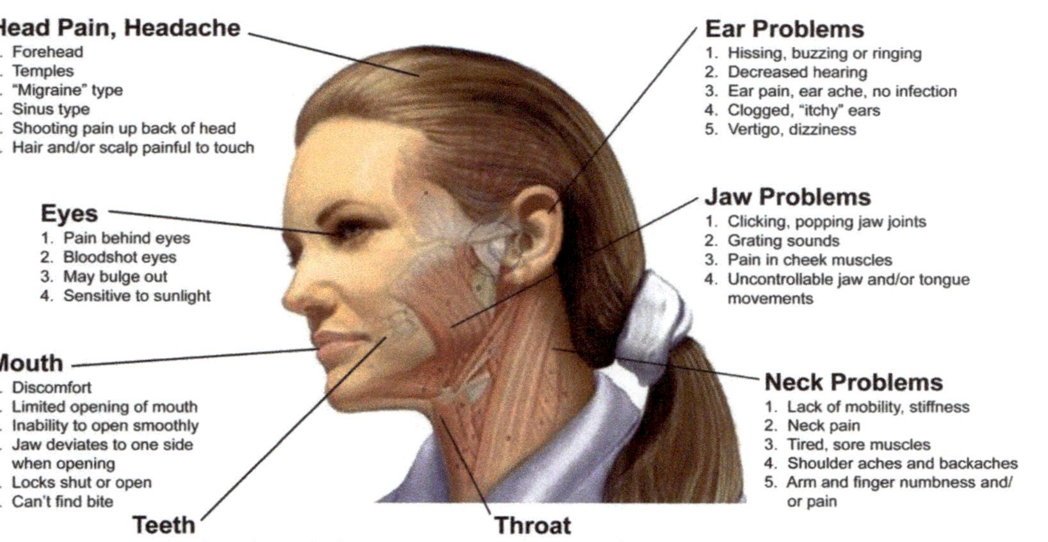

TMJ and the disk

The disk (in TMJ) is familiar to the ones in the knees, but these TMJ disks are different and more dynamic. The TMJ has several ligaments, bands and connective structures to keep it in place and movement.

Take care of your lower jaw movement. Do not overstretch it, by opening the mouth too far and/or too long. Be nice to yourself and all the body parts.

TMJ and Atlas correction

Channel on relation Atlas correction and TMJ

Atlas correction is coming from a disorder itself. It is caused by generations exposure to "other" energies for control until 2012. It had already no function anymore, but was resident in DNA. It caused body unbalances and pains. It needed to be corrected and as you know body unbalances can unbalance jaws and teeth, and so cause TMD. It was an unbalance between left and right. So yes, there might be effect. Is there a strong drect relation from neck to TMJ? No, and opposite is it possible to influence the Atlas by jaws, TMJ or teeth? Could be, but is in personal situations. Yes, also when you correct the Atlas it can influence the jaws and TMJ. This is stronger, because the Atlas disorder has been in the body for a long time, influencing posture and muscles. Everything has to adapt again, like a reset. Yes, Feldenkrais practices can Hlep in That. Enjoy finishing your book, we are excited!

Stress and TMJ

Depending on what you see as stress, there is a relation
between stress and TMJ. First of all, stress and fight flight
mode hormones make the body and muscles extra alert.
Secondly, you are in that mode less conscious on what
happens in and around the body and your habits go on
automatic pilot. Long term stress is not good at all for the
body.

Skull breathing

The skull bones/plates are flexible movable by the joints
between the plates. The skull has kind of breathing rhythm,
contracting fore and behind, so the skull widens to left and
right. This is caused by the inner fluids in the skull.

The flexibility is also necessary for protecting the brain and
glands inside from pressure and sudden outside forces, like
from an accident. This natural rhythm can be influenced or
blocked by TMJ, muscle stress etc, which can cause head
and neck pain. Pain is blocking or resisting natural rhythm
energy.

All body parts with joints needs movement, based on
rhythm.

Direct influence of organs by TMJ disorders

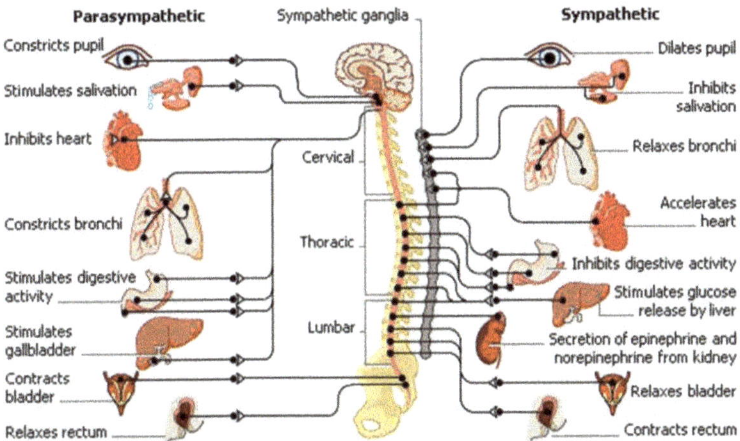

Following organs/energy fields are most influenced by
TMD:

- Lungs, nose, aspiration systems
- Digestion, stomach, liver, gallbladder
- Balance of male and female energies
- Diaphragm
- Heart

The TMJ muscles are influenced by thoughts and behaviour
in life. The muscles are very active, all day and maybe night.
The muscles are always working during talking, writing,
thinking and channeling. And maybe during dreams as
well. A lot of information, emotions from those activities
can stay stored in those muscles and cause stress. Not
spoken issues are very common to stay there, until they are
released.

Channel about what is the cause of TMJ/TMD

Greetings. I come to you with info on your called TMJ or earth rotating movement part. Do you understand? No? It is the part which connects you to your earth vessel for movement on earth. The joint is essential in all your movements, not only walking, talking or eating. You already know the physical muscle connections to your body, but you also breath and yes, breathing through nose is moving the muscles and jaws too, as reflex because you can also breath through your mouth. Is that better or worse? Neither. But the system is designed for nose breathing. You noticed that your jaw muscles also move during thinking or as a now writing. That's communicating! So, what is the problem for misaligning? Yes, you guess right, not being aligned. The human body and spirit are out of synchronization(sync) and then you are compensating and that hurts. But you cannot find another way in that moment.

Is it true that tonsils are damaged by mouth breathing? Not directly. Question yourself why you are mouth breathing. Nose blockage? Then why is that part infected? So, you see all the lines and sequences of a problem. Scroll back and you know the cause. So, healing of a displaced joint can by your "RVH", if you see the picture and how it should be. In your case many inverted parts (jaws, teeth, tonsils, head, muscles, neck, etc. Let me tell you the complete story. The neck is for head balancing. That is not, so phase one. The head parts are out of line, phase 2. From this start point you can go on. TMJ is not a disease by a virus, but behaviour, pressure, feeling unworthy, etc. Society problem for you tall guys. You wanted to be tall, but it has some troubles. Let me adjust some, sit straight.

It is working and resetting, trust it!

Second part of channel will come to you now. Hello Hans. TMJ/ TMD is not the only thing. The main stress is the smaller head (and higher). That is not only caused by bracelets. It has to do with escaping wide duality, left-right. That pressure is making you small. Relax that with compassion. Duality is not hurting. Emotions and feelings can be, if not mastered.

As young boy you hated that duality. Can we soften that for you now? **Yes please!** *That was old stuff you had not planned (you thought) in this life. Duality from higher perspective is beautiful magnetic energy(consciousness). It is in the moment experience. You wanted to go forward only. So, let us stop that together right. Yes, a little sad feeling now......It will pass, I already saw your smile.* **Thanks**. *You are welcome my son! Enjoy it and see you in other* **moments***!*

There is much more about TMJ and TMD, but with this basic info it is possible to change things in your life, when you are confronted with TMD. Follow first the basic steps about postures, position of jaws, tongue and specific about the breathing.

Healing

In this chapter I explain more about some possibilities for healing and some experiences with my clients.

The body is capable of healing, but we have to instruct and help the body to do it. This can be done by being aware of body expressions and happenings in your life and thoughts. One of the basics to help the body is breathing in the right way and the food intake.

For healing bad food habits, change diet and remove toxifications.

- Balance the phytic acid and remove toxification and remove all additions from your system, mainly the brain part.

- Check if Calcium and Phosphor are in balance in your system or you can have overshoot or shortage. With overshoot check your hormone systems and Glands (pituitary and Hypothalamus) Check if there are issues on the not absorbing of Calcium and or Phosphor.

- Check also the working of Parotid gland and Tonsils (Tonsil ring) and all interactions with the Hypothalamus.

- When hormones are out of balance adjust your diet and remove issues on that subject.

- The body is capable of healing and reconstructing itself. Check what blocks your healing.

Every tooth has its own donut energy field, including all blueprint info, and its own consciousness. In and with that energy field we can heal, recreate broken teeth or create new teeth. As mentioned before teeth are alive and are a part of you. So, treat them with respect and give them full support in attention, energy and the right food ingredients. If there is a bigger problem the tooth wants to express something very clear to you.

Channel about healing teeth

How can I heal broken teeth of client and myself? Broken teeth have meanings, which you can find out. In fact, there is already a scratch, breakline for a longer periode, which was not healed earlier. When it is "too" late or the "right moment" it will break down. What was the long separation which needs new energy? The scratch is facing surface, so you can build on the remaining basics. So, what was the part that needed to be separated? Can we grow teeth parts back? Yes. There is a fundament? Yes, and it is alive, always, even if it seems not to you and your dentist. Be aware to make the fundament strong, alive and let it be a part of you. No separation anymore.

So, what about to do about it with the client? Let it rest for a while, keep it clean with water and nourish your nerves at that surface point. To heal it you need building blocks. The will to be complete and ok with that missing part in your life and to fill it up with something different, equal but without that "break" energy.

That's the one!

Then face the part left in the jaw and be one with it, accept the you, also that part of you.

Technical you can build it up again with the right components and the right energy with that tooth. Ask for guidance in such a process. You can do for your issues and for the client, but she is not ready yet, and you have to find out.

You are not ready yet, first clean more in your emotions and systems and hidden thoughts about it. Find the cracks and very old issues about this "material" healing. It is done with vortex healing like we told you before. The vortex is on the spot for "creating" materials, but you don't believe that.

Take a while to see this in meditation in that place(tooth), you will be guided.

Go to the spot where changes should be made. You will see a cleaned and clean your believes on what you see.

Good luck, have fun, syl.

Following channel came during other channel, just before I had to do a healing session.

Channel about teeth healing on pregnant women.

What about tooth treatment on pregnant women? (I was already in conversation) The woman is referring to treatments with fillings, chemicals and other stuff on teeth. The teeth area is very sensitive and very fast absorbed by the blood. These chemicals are directly in all systems and the brain of the fetus. Young children are very sensitive in the mouth and head, so the resist all chemicals and food from their nature if they want. Grown up can have more poison and strange tastes in their mouth, because the mouth is less sensitive. So, stop all those teeth treatments 3 months before pregnancy to keep the body clean for the pregnancy and the health of the baby.

Meridians connections to teeth

Herewith the connections of the meridians to the teeth as I discovered it. I know there are many charts on internet with connections to organs, body parts and emotions. But as mentioned before, there is much more than only meridians. Meridian info can be helpful, but the bigger picture from holistic view is the most important information to know what and why. In my practise I use the unique teeth numbers 1-32 instead of the 4x8 numbers. This to be clear and no mistakes about upper, lower, left or right. See picture below.

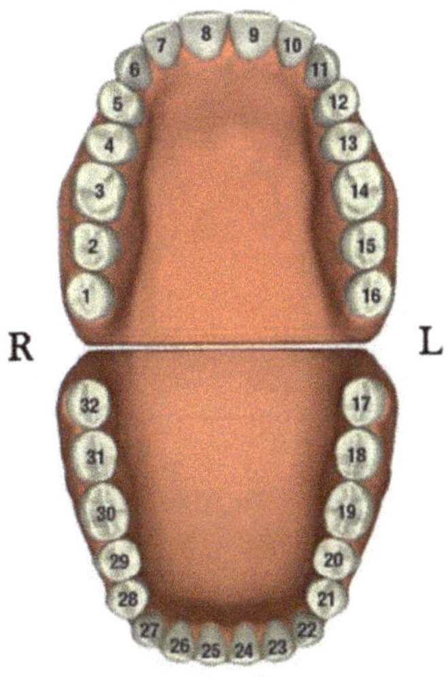

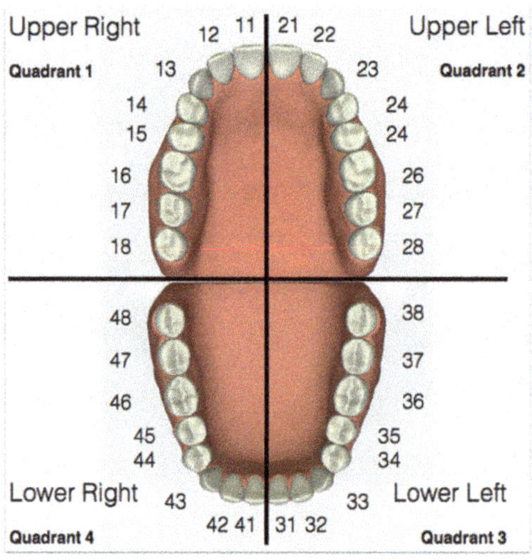

Upper Right
Quadrant 1
Upper Left
Quadrant 2
12 11 21 22
13 23
14 24
15 24
16 26
17 27
18 28
48 38
47 37
46 36
45 35
44 34
Lower Right
Quadrant 4
Lower Left
Quadrant 3
43 33
42 41 31 32

Meridian chart:

Name		Energy	Body	L/R	Teeth
Lung	LU	Out	Hand	R	19,20
				L	29,30
Large Intestine	LI	In	Hand	R	12,18,19
				L	05,30
Stomach	ST	Out	Foot	R	19,20,21
				L	29,30
Spleen (Pancreas)	SP	In	Foot	R	29,04
				L	13,20
Heart	HT	Out	Hand	R	01
				L	16
Small Intestine	SI	In	Hand	R	14,15
				L	02,03
Bladder	BL	Out	Foot	R	11
				L	06
Kidney	KI	In	Foot	R	25,26
				L	22,23
Heart Constrictor	HC	Out	Hand	R	15,18
				L	02,31,32
Tripple warmer	TH	In	Hand	R	20,21
				L	Lower Jaw Right
Gall Bladder	GB	Out	Foot	R	09,10,11,20,21,22,23,24
				L	06.07,08,25,26,27,28
Liver	LI	In	Foot	R	30,31
				L	02
Governing	GV	To Top	Back		06,07,08,09,10,11,12
Central	CV	To Top	Front		20,21,22,23,24,25,26,27,28

Healing Examples

Some examples from my practise, where I helped people on following subjects:

- Remove inflammation pains.

- Release tooth pains.

- Explained to clients why tooths were lost, damaged, etc.

- Worked with clients with overall problems in the mouth, like many cavities, gum problems, etc.

- Explained, by info from the tooth, what had to be changed in life, their thinking and actions.

- Made clear that the damaged tooth was not the problem, but neighbour teeth or the tooth in the other jaw.

- Release of stress, caused by implants.

- Release of stress of the jaw/face muscles.

- Etc.

Literature

Moshe Feldenkrais	Awareness through movement
	Body & Mature Behavior
	The Potent Self
Robert Kulacz & Thomas E. Levy	The roots of disease
Ken Southward	A hypothetical role for vitamin K2 in the endocrine and exocrine aspects of dental caries
	Wisdom teeth dental scam & why you need your wisdom teeth
	Acumeridian understanding of organ systems and emotions
	The systemic theory of dental caries
	Wellness dentistry-the big wave
Wieger Veerman	Euritmie
Dirk Schreckenbach	Zahngeflüster
	Die Zähne, Spiegelbild deiner Seele
Tsao Hsueh-Lien and Bruce Thornton	Meridians
George T.J. Huang	Dental pulp and dentin tissue engineering andregeneration
Weston A. Price	Nutrition and Physical Degeneration Link: http://gutenberg.net.au/ebooks02/0200251h.html#toc
Kate Evans Scott	The Natural Cure for Tooth decay
Ramiel Nagel	Cure Tooth decay (with nutrition)
	Cure Gum disease naturally
Catherine Shanahan	Deep Nutrition
John Nicholles	The Teeth in relation to Beauty, Voice and Health

Ensanya Ali Abou Neel (and others)	Tissue Engineering in Dentistry
John E. Upledger	Cell Talk
Dr Wolfgang Kuhl	Heal your Teeth
Nadine Artemis	Holistic Dental Care
Michel Montaud	Nos Dents une porte vers la santé
	De la dent à l'homme, un parcours bouleversant
Ralph Steinman DDS MS, John Leonora PhD	Dentinal Fluid Transport
Michèle Caffin	Als tanden konden kiezen
Cynthia Peterson, PT	The TMJ Healing Plan
S. Kent Lauson, DDS, MS, Orthodontist	Straight talk about crooked teeth
Marco Bischof	Biophotonen, Das Licht in unseren Zellen
Dr. Gerald Jahl/ Dr. Viviane Osterreicher/ Dr. Gernot osterreicher	Osterreich auf den Zahn gefühlt
Dr. Ulrich Volz/ Dr. Hauke Heinzel u.a.	Zähne gut – alles gut
von Keng und Machang Sanga	The war in your teeth

www.ingramcontent.com/pod-product-compliance
Lightning Source LLC
LaVergne TN
LVHW051109180726
843512LV00011B/775